School-Parent Collaboration
in Indigenous Communities

Iris Manor-Binyamini

School-Parent Collaborations in Indigenous Communities

Providing Services for Children with Disabilities

Springer

Iris Manor-Binyamini
Department of Special Education
University of Haifa
Haifa, Israel

ISBN 978-1-4939-4373-9   ISBN 978-1-4614-8984-9 (eBook)
DOI 10.1007/978-1-4614-8984-9
Springer New York Heidelberg Dordrecht London

Printed on acid-free paper

Springer is part of Springer Science+Business Media (www.springer.com)

*To my parents, Michael (of blessed memory)
and Noga Manor*

To my husband and children

*Without your support this book would not
have been written*

"Inspiration, whatever its nature, is born of a perpetual 'I don't know'. Any knowledge that doesn't give rise to new questions quickly expires: it lacks the vital warmth that sustains life" (Wisława Szymborska, In Praise of Dreams. Tel Aviv: Attention to Poetry 2004, page 163).

I sincerely hope that this book raises many questions for readers, thus ensuring that this important issue does not expire quickly or lose its vital sustenance.

Preface

Indigenous peoples across the world have other stories to tell (Smith L.T., 1999)

Indigenous people are just as much a part of the complex modern world as any of us; they may be different, they may be unique, but they must be nurtured, respected, and allowed to emerge. This is particularly pertinent in regard to children with disabilities, in light of the fact that worldwide, minorities are overrepresented in populations of people with disabilities. In some areas of the world, the disability rate among indigenous peoples is more than double the rate in the non-indigenous population (see Chap. 2 for specific data). Indigenous populations collaborating with the parents of children with disabilities are a prerequisite for treatment to prove effective; hence, the subject of this book is of paramount importance.

There are seven chapters in the book, some informative and some practicable. Chapters 1–4 provide the background, bringing the reader up to date on the relevant professional literature and terminology, and review the current state of several indigenous communities worldwide. Chapters 5–7 take an in-depth look, through the case studies presented, at the Bedouin community in the Negev desert in Israel, and examine the collaboration between professionals and parents of children with disabilities in this community. The following is a detailed description of the chapters in the book.

Chapter 1

The first chapter, which opens the book, is the backdrop for the entire book; in this chapter, I present the common characteristics unique to indigenous communities and to children with disabilities in these communities. It opens with a definition of indigenous peoples, and presents the world's indigenous population numbering about 257–350 million people. Later in the chapter, I survey the attempt to explain the source of the difficulties and challenges common to all indigenous communities around the world; these include high frequency of health risks, elevated school dropout rates, child labor, the need for more extensive support services, a lack of financial resources and the resulting condition of perpetual poverty, and subjection to acts of dispossession and spirit-breaking.

The second part of the chapter, titled Indigenous Communities and Children with Disabilities in the World, examines the concept of *disability* and the problematic nature of the definition, and then focuses on children with disabilities in indigenous communities, more specifically, the issue of precisely documenting their numbers, the fact that it is nevertheless known that the rates of children with disabilities in the indigenous communities are extraordinarily high. Some explanatory factors are suggested and the topic of support services is broached.

The work of preparing the first chapter was like assembling a mosaic: gathering information from all over the world, in an attempt to produce a representative image. Unfortunately, the image presented here is still only partial. This is due to the absence of data and the incomplete nature of the data available in the existing literature and research reports. Furthermore, there is also a certain bias in the data. Remote locations and language barriers have made it logistically difficult to include indigenous areas in major surveys; and even when indigenous peoples are included in surveys, the resulting disaggregated data are rarely used to reflect their particular conditions.

We know least about the regions with the largest estimated indigenous populations: for example, there is a dearth of accurate demographic and health data from Africa, China, South Asia, and the Former Soviet Union. Despite these gaps of information, there is much evidence about the situation of indigenous peoples in Canada, the USA, Australia, and New Zealand, and to a lesser extent, Latin America. Even in this nation, most studies show an alarming situation.

In order to deal with the lack of data or the partial data, I chose to structure the review as a mosaic, namely, by providing concrete examples so as to illustrate the topics I discuss, each time presenting a different country/countries, with the available existing data. In addition, the purpose of the dichotomous presentation of the subtopics in this first chapter was to provide as wide an overview as possible of indigenous communities around the world and the difficult reality with which they must contend, a reality in which it is often impossible to discern the various characteristics of the indigenous group, as they are so intricately related. Thus, for example, there is an indifferentiable connection between poverty, health conditions, and lack of education.

Given that the study of indigenous populations is conducted both globally and locally, I had to read a wide variety of materials from a wide variety of countries. This is one of the book's advantages, yet it is also a disadvantage. Due to the fact that most of the existing material is in English, there is a disproportionate representation of materials written about indigenous communities in English-speaking countries. However, since English-language texts are an important means of communication among those who study and represent indigenous issues in different countries, this literature is likely to play an important role in the understanding of indigenous psychologies.

Chapter 2

This chapter presents concepts that are crucial to understanding how indigenous parents view disability. Understanding the concept of "culture," for instance, enables us to understand how indigenous communities differ in their conceptualization of disability, and the perspective, understanding, and expectations with which parents of children with disabilities approach collaboration with professionals in school. The concepts that will be discussed in this chapter are *culture, lands and territories, indigenous knowledge*, and *indigenous psychology*.

The prism through which I chose to address the concepts in this chapter is educational (rather than judicial, anthropological, medical, sociological, or based on any other discipline that deals with this domain). Hence, these concepts, which were selected out of a wide range of concepts that could be examined when dealing with indigenous communities, are those which enable the (lay) reader, as well as the professional, to understand the concept of disability from the perspective of indigenous peoples, and to take into account the beliefs, perceptions, values, context, and history that parents of children with disabilities bring with them into a collaboration with professionals at the school. The argument enfolded into this chapter (and book) is that there is something universal in the phenomenon of indigenous peoples as a group, and specifically on the topic of children with disabilities and parents of children with disabilities in indigenous communities.

In addition, it is important to note that there are many difficulties regarding the issue of conceptualization: almost every key concept introduced in this book, such as *indigenous*, and *culture*, has many possible definitions, and some of the concepts, such as the concept of *indigenous psychology*, are subject to disagreement in the professional literature.

Chapter 3

This chapter, titled School Professionals and Parents of Children with Disabilities, first introduces the importance of the school and the benefits of a multidisciplinary team, and includes a detailed description of a research study that aimed to locate indigenous (Bedouin) children with disabilities living in tents. Then the chapter takes a close look at the parents of children with disabilities and the act of parenting and considers psychological models of parents' reactions to a child's disability, and finally contemplates the roles of the professionals and parents in special educational schools.

This chapter (like the entire book) focuses on parents of children and adolescents of ages 3–21, in the context of educational systems in the State of Israel, which, like in other Western countries, provide support services and give care to children of these ages, in special education kindergarten and schools. The book does not deal with adults, that is, people with disabilities older than 21; dealing with adults with disabilities of these age requires focusing on different issues altogether, such as employment, quality of life, independence, integration in the community and society, and so on. This required another book.

Chapter 4

The first part of the chapter discusses collaboration between parents of children with disabilities and professionals in schools, which encompasses the following issues: definition of the term *collaboration*, characteristics of collaboration with culturally and linguistically diverse (CLD) parents of children with disabilities at school, effective collaboration between professionals and parents of children with disabilities at special education schools, and collaboration between professionals and parents in indigenous communities. The second part of the chapter presents a study that reveals the dimensions of collaboration between professionals and parents in a special education school in a Western country.

Chapter 5

This chapter is divided into two parts: the first part focuses on the background of the Bedouin community in the Negev desert, that is, the characteristics unique to the Bedouin community, while the second part examines the characteristics, the challenges, and the difficulties that the Bedouin community shares with other indigenous communities. This last part is based on the first chapter of this book, which considered the characteristics that indigenous communities around the world have in common.

Chapter 6

This chapter presents a situation report on children with disabilities in the Bedouin community and a review of the conditions and functioning of the special education framework available to the Bedouin community in southern Israeli's Negev region.

Chapter 7

In this chapter I have sought to give voice to the Bedouin professionals working with children with disabilities, as well as to Bedouin parents of children with disabilities, whose voices are not heard in the existing research, and to try to understand their perceptions and the ways in which they comprehend and define parenting and the concept and the practice of collaboration in the school.

This chapter concludes with a section in which I suggest principles of indigenously inclined collaboration derived from the chapters of the book and the case study discussed in the previous part of this chapter. These principles can be used as a springboard for discussion. At the same time, they provide a backdrop from which to formulate new questions in a way that increases our understanding and our capacity to provide the best possible bridge to collaboration. Each of the principles is presented in an identical manner, referring to three elements: the subject that the principle addresses, the goal of the principle, and the assumptions behind it.

Chapters 6 and 7 are based on studies that I conducted during my postdoctoral work. The study was funded by two different sources: the Shalem Foundation and the Arno Center for the Study of the Bedouin community.

I hope that the readers of this book come away with a better understanding of this complex subject, the collaboration between professionals and parents of children with disabilities in indigenous communities, and find in it a resource for developing and promoting this type of collaboration.

My greatest wish is that this book will in some small way contribute to the work of a variety of people involved with the population of children with disabilities and their parents in indigenous communities worldwide, namely, students, researchers, and/or professionals of various disciplines—education, special education, psychology, medicine, social work, health, welfare, anthropology—as well to policy makers and those who implement the intervention, by inspiring them to introduce future improvements in the education and services intended for and children with disabilities and their parents in indigenous communities.

In Lieu of an Opening Statement

Salma's story*

Salma takes a deep breath, and starts speaking.

Having a child with disabilities in the Bedouin community is a crisis, an irregular event; it can either bring the family closer together or tear it apart. The first step is shock, denial, anger, that's what the men feel toward their wives—"damn this defect that she gave birth to…." They turn their anger toward the woman, sometimes the women get a beating. There is guilt—"maybe this son will not be useful to the community." Having a son brings power to the tribe, to the family in the Bedouin community, but this one won't be useful to the community. Having a daughter detracts from the honor of the family, she will be used. That is the worst thing that can happen to the ego of a Bedouin. You can see the women are depressed, a woman has, on average, six or seven more children; she spends 24 h a day taking care of them, and so a child like this, it's twice as hard; the woman gets burnt out, exhausted, she might collapse, and this takes its toll. You see women letting themselves go, becoming distant, like there is something wrong with them.

She looks at me.

You have to understand, it's shameful having a damaged child. You hide it, sometimes you don't take it to get treatments, and this is true for boys and for girls. It can also cause conflicts between partners, the child's parents, if there are other damaged children in the family. The blame is pointed toward her (meaning the mother), many times the man will leave, especially if the women had more than one damaged child. The first year is of critical importance, the man might desert the family, or he might take care of the family and become a part of those caring for the child. I am referring to weaker populations, people who end up on welfare, asking for assistance. There is a lot of difficulty in handling the day-to-day tasks and caring for the child. Mostly it's the woman who does the caring, and this kind of child needs a lot of care. Sometimes the man participates, you have to get out of the house and drive all the way to the Child Development Center, to the hospital… a woman can only go by car if a man is with her, so either they both go or it's just the man, and the woman doesn't get to go at all. Another problem is the issue of accessibility: we see

xv

a lot of problems, it has to do with the family's financial situation, it's easier if they own a car, but if they don't and they live far away from a road, then the woman has to walk and drag the child with her, and then you just have to pray that she has a repayment guarantee, because if she gets all the way to the Child Development Center and they won't treat the child because she can't produce the document displaying the health maintenance organization's repayment guarantee, then the next time she just won't go. If she leaves the house, she has to arrange for someone to stay with the other children. This week we had a call where an 8-year-old girl had to stay and babysit for three babies because the mother had to go to the hospital with another child, and that is the best case scenario.

She is silent…

Many of the families live on a social security budget. If the father works, many times if this kind of a child is born, the father will stop working, and you have to keep in mind that it's very difficult to find work to begin with; there isn't an option for a half-time position, because many of them have no training or experience whatsoever. These are tragedies; the entire arrangement of the family's life revolves around the care of this one child, the quality of life of the whole family is decreased. Facing the welfare offices is just another incident that degrades the man's sense of honor. Regarding rights, most of our families are illiterate, so when they go to the market, the bank, and the employment office once a month, they have difficulty getting by. They leave the house about four times a month. If a child have a disability is, that child has rights, and in most cases, the family is unaware of that, of what these children deserve: a disability allowance, travel reimbursements… if they have no guidance or knowledge, their situation gets worse, and they might stop caring for the child. Mothers just give up.

There are also difficulties when facing the outside world—the difficulties that families go through when dealing with the authorities "it's just like landing on the moon," social security, education… think of a Bedouin man, no education, no skills, suddenly he has to argue, to communicate with the various authorities. He is a parent who doesn't have the skills of the professionals, and then add to that his emotions and his defense mechanisms. With all this, he must find the strength to fight for the child's rights, but he's exhausted, and so he takes his anger out on the professionals. The father isn't angry at me, the professional, the social worker; he's projecting his feelings, his anger at himself, at the situation. Remember that these children stay at home from birth until they turn 5 years old, because there is no educational framework for this age group, and these are crucial ages in terms of development, adding to the burden and hardships that the mother has to deal with. Sometimes there is an educational framework, but it's not suitable for the child, for his needs. Nowadays, all of the educational frameworks are rehabilitative kindergartens, and they let in autistic children and those with mental retardation. Sometimes parents, even if they are not educated, see children who do not fit their child's behavior, and prefer to keep their own child at home. There is also a lot of free time, even if the child is in an educational framework, there is no long school day, where the children stay at school till 5 p.m., even if there are educational frameworks at—(mentions the name of a distant town), who is going to arrange transportation for these children? Families, because of the conditions, sometimes, *wiping a tear, tie up their child, to prevent him from hurting himself, because the* *child can go to the wadi and fall in, so they use ropes, pegs, sometimes chains, to tie* *up their child. Now, as the child gets older, it becomes more difficult to deal with* *this situation. This age is particularly problematic for girls.* She is silent, her eyes turned toward the floor. *We see girls, especially if they're pretty, sexual developed,* *from the age of 12, there is concern for the girl's safety. If the girl is developed, the* *parents are afraid and so they stop sending her to school. They wouldn't admit this* *at the transportation system, but they drive the children without a chaperon. The* *parents would prefer to have the girl in a framework outside of the home.* She is silent... *I never thought that a Bedouin family would remove a child from the home,* *but there is no other choice. And what do you do when the girl reaches the age of 18* *Let's call it "a marriage of rehabilitation," meant to protect the girl and the disabled* *boy, so that the woman won't be left alone, lonely. They reach a state where they* *marry off the retarded with the retarded, and there is a rehabilitative aspect to this* *act. For men, it's easier if you bring them a beautiful, healthy bride.* She is silent, breaths in... *Some healthy women feel that it is better to marry a man with mild* *retardation than to be a second wife. The men often get their way about this. I never* *saw a woman with mild mental retardation who was married off, but men with mild* *mental retardation—I have. If they do marry off a woman with mild mental retarda-* *tion, it would be to an old widower or someone who already has three old wives.* *The old man gets someone to take care of him; the young girl doesn't end up getting* *used. At best, she might give birth to a healthy child. She will have a child, and when* *she is older, the child will look after her. Many times, she ends up being a project* *for the other wives, and they have to take care of her, help her, guide her. That's* *mental retardation, they hide mental health issues and behavioral problems; these* *days they ask and inquire about the woman before the wedding; it wasn't like this in* *the past—they never saw, never met the woman beforehand, and many times they* *wouldn't throw her out, they would just take a second wife, if the first one is dis-* *abled. Damaged girls usually come from farther away, not from the south, and then* *after a few weeks, everything comes to a head and the conflicts start.*

But there are also successes, and that's what keeps me going and allows me to *get up every morning to do this work.*

She smiles.

I'll give you one example, to represent what we go through with the families: *I met a boy on the street, 13 years old, crawling on the road. I saw him, we got out* *of the car and decided to talk to him, he spoke well and to the point, he pointed to* *his house, and we decided to go in, even though he wasn't in our care. Luckily, the* *mother and grandmother were home, the grandmother is the mother's cousin. They* *said he wasn't in any framework, a 13 year old boy that has never been in any edu-* *cational framework, not getting any help from the Social Security Institute, no medi-* *cal help, neglected, crooked arms... it was clear that this whole family needed to be* *the focus and not just the child. It turned out that because of this child, the father* *gradually left the home; it was under the wire, because he only came to sleep at the* *house. He married a second wife and then he even he stopped sleeping at home, and they had no source of income, and seven children; the grandmother took care of them, only gave them food. The grandmother and the mother could not help, so I decided to turn to the father. It's a risk, because it means reopening old conflicts. When I talked to the father, I thought he'd throw me out of the house. Apparently, he was waiting for us to talk with him. He told me he'd do anything I asked, and then he handled matters; the child started seeing a doctor regularly, received a wheel-chair, income support, they built a shed with this money. The success was thanks to the father... I will not tell you the whole story, but today he is a social activist...*

Salma's (pseudonym) words, with which this book opens, were spoken during an interview I conducted with her in 2009. Salma's words give voice to the everyday life of parents and children with disabilities in an indigenous community—the Bedouin community in the Negev desert in Israel. Based on research information, this book attempts to give voice to parents and experts in indigenous populations around the world.

Researcher's voice
Researching the topic presented in this book, the collaboration between profession-als and parents of children with disabilities in the indigenous community of Bedouins in Israel was for me a triple challenge: there I was, a secular Jewish female research-ing a cultural different from mine in terms of language, religion, culture, and gender hierarchy. This long-term study that I conducted, as well as other studies that I am currently conducting in the Bedouin community in the Negev, created many internal conflicts for me as a researcher: I had many questions, doubts, and dilemmas, due to the differences between myself as a researcher and the participants, and due to the primary nature of the study. Entering an unmapped territory meant working alone, given that even the latest research literature provided only partial answers to the questions that arose. In regard to the personal and interpersonal processes experienced by a solitary scholar in an indigenous community, there were no answers at all. Over the years of continuous research, this study has summoned for me numerous and varied dilemmas, such as how does a researcher create trust in a gated community, such as the Bedouin community, especially on the case of primal research? How does one deal with gender aspects such as a cultural resis-tance to having a woman interview men? What does a researcher do with sensitive research materials that may cause the participants harm if published? How does a researcher deal with the emotional aspects that the research topic evokes, and does a sensitive research topic affect the research and the writing? How does one deal with ethical dilemmas that arise in the research field? How does a researcher rec-oncile a narrative that she was told when it is not consistent with her own profes-sional and scholarly worldview? Over years of research, I have managed to find answers to every dilemma that has come up; however, this book does not contain these answers. They are worthy of a book unto themselves.

Acknowledgments

To "my research subjects," the many parents, and professionals who led me through the labyrinths of their lives and their experiences with the special education system in the Bedouin community, my eternal gratitude. Each and every one of them, parents and professionals, has been my teacher, translator, and interpreter, each shedding light on the essence of their existence. Without their help and guidance, I would have proceeded blindly, trying to capture the reality of life of this community. I thank them for agreeing to open their hearts to me at all times; without their openness and willingness to share with me their experiences, good and bad, I would not have made my way through the physical and emotional challenges of this journey of research, nor could I have achieved the scientific insights that followed.

A special thank you to Othman Abu–Ajaj, who was the principal of the Kseifa School for Special Education during the period of research and is now the head of the Department of Society and Community in the Bedouin community in the Negev, for years of productive professional dialogue and support across borders and cultures.

I first arrived at the Bedouin community during my postdoctoral studies, which began in 2004 and lasted 3 years. Each of my scientific journeys, and particularly those to the unrecognized Bedouin settlements, was laden with intense emotional experiences. Although some of these experiences still remain unresolved, they increased my determination, and especially my desire to penetrate the veil of the "other" and understand the Bedouin community "from the inside."

Ever since I first met them, I have maintained contact with the professionals, the children, and the parents of children with disabilities, and this ongoing relationship is manifested in the reports and articles that I have written about the special education frameworks and ways in which parents and siblings of children with disabilities in this community cope with the related challenges. Looking back today at those 3 years of postdoctoral work, I get an overwhelming sense of helplessness, I recall the alienation and distancing that I experienced, which at the same time was combined with an inexplicable attraction and sense of belonging. At the time, I didn't know or understand that my academic life was already bound with the lives of the people of the community. The differences between the Bedouins and me, in appearance, language, and way of life, seemed infinite; yet, I found something in them—in their humanity—that spoke to me and has created a strong bond of existential significance.

In many ways, in the course of my research, the long-term stay in the field helped blur the boundaries that separated me from the Bedouins and attenuated the harsh distinctions that come with traditional hierarchies and power relationships, such as those between researcher and subjects, observer and observed, and stranger and insider. Nonetheless, I was and still am a white woman working among Bedouins of darker complexion, a Jewish woman among Muslims, a Western-educated woman facing a complex network of a different world of knowledge characterized by principles and logic which sometimes were clear to me, but in many other cases seemed foreign and strange. Often, in moments of pain, sadness, and frustration, I found myself still thinking in Western terms. Every time these thoughts came up, I would get angry at myself, and yet, during this journey of research I repeatedly encountered situations and experiences that contrasted sharply with my understandings, my knowledge, and my most basic personal and professional beliefs. I found myself in constant dialogue with myself whenever I saw parents of children with intellectual disabilities tying up their child with iron chains, when I saw a Bedouin mother carrying her adolescent son, with cerebral palsy, on her back for many miles in the 40 °C desert heat, or every time I heard "religious" explanations and "cultural" justifications for the murder of a relative over a blood feud. The decision to anchor my questions in systematic research stemmed from my great interest in the subject, of course, as well as from a desire to be able—after years spent in research—to translate "objective" observations into a voice, an insight, and from my determination to present in the public arena an analysis of this reality that might reach public consciousness.

The experts and the parents of children with disabilities who participated in the studies presented in this book are, in the words of one educator at a special education school, "*the people who protect the candle's flame in the dark*," people who despite the complex, difficult, and sometimes impossible reality they face, continue fighting every day and every hour for the lives and the quality of life of children with disabilities in the Bedouin community.

This book is dedicated to them, with great appreciation and love.

I owe another thank you to two women whose help and support hopefully have made this book clearer—to Lee Cornfield, the editor of the book, for finding the right and most accurate words for the ideas that I wanted to express throughout the book, and to Rella Kurtser, for her wonderful ability to turn my ideas into clear and comprehensible diagrams, with never ending patience.

University of Haifa, Haifa, Israel   Iris Manor-Binyamini

About the Author

Dr. Iris Manor-Binyamini is a Lecturer and a senior faculty member of the Department of Special Education at the University of Haifa in Israel. Her academic interests include special education in the Bedouin community in Israel, inter- and intra-community comparisons of the coping styles and strategies used by parents and siblings of adults with various disabilities and from different minority communities in Israel (the Bedouin, Druze, and Ultraorthodox Jewish communities), and the collaboration within multi-disciplinary teams in special education schools, as well as the collaboration between these teams and the parents of children with disabilities.

One of her recent publications, Parental Coping with Developmental Disorders in Adolescents within the Ultraorthodox Jewish Community in Israel, published in 2012 in the *Journal of Autism and Developmental Disorders*, was recognized by the Psychology Progress team as a Key Research Article in Psychology.

Dr. Manor-Binyamini has written extensively on the Psychology of the Bedouin Community, including a comprehensive research evaluation report: Assessing a Multidisciplinary Training Program for Professionals Working with Children with Special Needs in the Bedouin Community.

Contents

Part I
Theory

Chapter 1
Indigenous Communities and Children with Disabilities in the World: Unique Characteristics of Indigenous Communities and Children with Disabilities

1.1 Overview

The Declaration on the Rights of Indigenous Peoples was adopted by the UN General Assembly on Thursday, 13 September 2007, by a majority of 144 states in favor, with 4 votes against and 11 abstentions. During the Durban Review Conference in April 2009, 182 states from all regions of the world reached consensus on an outcome document in which they "*Welcome[d]* the adoption of the UN Declaration on the Rights of Indigenous Peoples, which has a positive impact on the protection of victims and, in this context, urge[d] states to take all necessary measures to implement the rights of indigenous peoples in accordance with international human rights instruments without discrimination…" (UN Office of the High Commissioner for Human Rights, *Outcome Document of the Durban Review Conference*, 24 April 2009, para. 73).

The change in policy towards indigenous peoples and communities as manifested in the declaration of rights has led primarily to the process of democratization in some countries and to the establishment of an indigenous peoples' organization within the UN. The following describes in brief the main developments in the UN's policy on this issue.

In 1957, the development and integration of these populations was discussed and the first covenant regarding indigenous populations was accepted by the UN; in 1982, the Working Group on Indigenous Populations (WGIP) was established; in 1993, the UN General Assembly ratified a draft of the Declaration on the Rights of Indigenous Peoples; in 2002, a permanent forum on indigenous issues was established, which has been active since and still produces current updated reports (in 2013); and in 2007, after a 25-year process, the Declaration on the Rights of Indigenous Peoples was adopted, anchoring the rights of indigenous peoples and protecting their lands, resources, and cultures. Although the declaration does not comprehensively bind the UN member states, it does establish clear norms that delineate the desired attitude towards indigenous peoples. Thus, the development of the UN policy towards indigenous peoples may be perceived as dynamic rather than

I. Manor-Binyamini, *School-Parent Collaborations in Indigenous Communities: Providing Services for Children with Disabilities*, DOI 10.1007/978-1-4614-8984-9_1, © Springer Science+Business Media New York 2014

linear, and while significant shifts have taken place primarily in the courts, they have relied on changing trends in the public and political discourse.

The consolidation of the new approach was a result of fierce debates between the different interest groups. The collective rights of indigenous nations are anchored in a variety of arrangements, with some countries establishing their relations with their indigenous nations on the basis of agreements and contracts. An agreement may be specific and constitute one step in a reconciliation process. Another possible arrangement is to choose the legislative path, by formulating a "Charter of Rights," which is the approach that has been adopted in the United States, Canada, and New Zealand. Other measures leading towards deep-seated recognition include integrating the customary, native law with the prevailing or civil law; recognizing common ownership of resources such as land; establishing compensation by means of legislation that grants equal rights while admitting past mistakes and seeking forgiveness. This variety of approaches, as well as the evolving process of change, is made evident only by means of global comparative studies, which have documented policy and legal developments towards indigenous nations in various countries. While the declaration adopted by the UN does not dictate one universal definition of "indigenous peoples" to be agreed upon by all nations, it is nevertheless clear that at the international level, the definitions introduced by the UN's working group (WGIP) have been widely accepted (182 countries, as of 2009). Therefore, this is also the definition that will be used in this book. It is based on Cobo Martinez's definition from 1972, proposed at the UN General Assembly (see the UN site). According to this definition, indigenous nations are

- Communities that have a prior presence and use of a given space
- Communities with a unique cultural continuity—language, religion, tradition, economy, laws and institutions, and a will to continue to live separately as a collective
- Communities that have traditional societies, frequently half-nomadic/tribal
- Communities that identify themselves as a separate cultural group
- Communities whose members experienced a colonial intrusion and a history of exclusion, dispossession, conquest, forced cultural change, discrimination, and/ or displacement from their main living spaces by the modern state

In certain countries, however, these communities are not legally recognized as indigenous peoples. Given that in some countries the definition of indigenous peoples is controversial, each country defines these populations differently. I chose to use the UN's definition as the foundation for this book, since it offers a unified scale for defining indigenous communities worldwide. In addition to the lack of a universally accepted definition at the international level, there is also no agreement regarding the term "indigenous" itself.

Different countries use a variety of terms to refer to groups within their borders, which have been recognized by international legislation as "indigenous peoples." These designations include, among others, "Native Americans" and "Pacific Islanders" in the United States; "Inuit," "Metis," and "First Nation" in Canada; Aborigines in Australia; the Māori in New Zealand; Hill tribes in South East Asia;

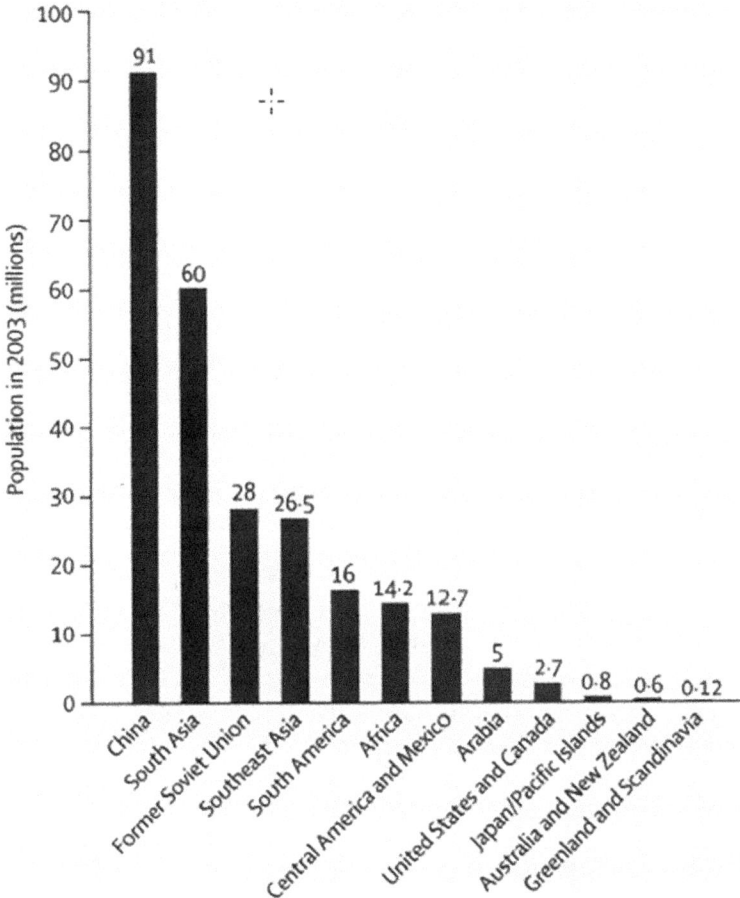

Fig. 1.1 Indigenous populations by region of the world (Adapted from Maybury-Lewis 2007)

indigenous ethnic minorities, Scheduled Tribes, or Adivasi, in India; tribal groups, autochthonous groups, or *minzoku*, in Japan; and the list goes on. As the variety of terms suggests, defining who is indigenous is a difficult task.

Due to the absence of a single and all-encompassing definition, there are very different demographic estimates of indigenous peoples. The latest figures from international nongovernmental organizations and from academia estimate that there are between 257 and 350 million indigenous people in the world today (see Fig. 1.1).

We know the least about regions with the largest estimated indigenous populations; for example, there is a dearth of accurate demographic and health-related data from Africa, China, South Asia, and the Former Soviet Union. The variance among these communities is manifest in several manners. For instance, contemporary distinct indigenous groups survive in populations ranging from only a few dozen to hundreds of thousands and more. Many indigenous populations have undergone a dramatic decline and even extinction and remain threatened in many parts of the world. Indigenous societies range from those that have been significantly exposed to the colonizing or expansionary activities of other societies (such as the Maya peoples of Mexico and Central America) to those who as yet remain relatively isolated from any external influence (such as the Sentinelese and Jarawa of the Andaman Islands). Some have also been assimilated by other populations or have undergone many other changes. In other cases, indigenous populations are undergoing a recovery or expansion in numbers.

Indigenous societies may be settled in a given locale or region, or they may exhibit a nomadic lifestyle across a large territory; generally, however, they are associated historically with a specific territory, on which they depend for their livelihood. Indigenous societies are found in every inhabited climate zone and continent of the world.

Despite the lack of a universally agreed upon definition and term, there are difficulties and challenges that are common to all indigenous communities in the world. The following section highlights some of the challenges and difficulties that indigenous children encounter, regardless of their geographic location.

1.1.1 High Frequency of Health Risks

In December 1993, the United Nations General Assembly proclaimed the International Decade of the World's Indigenous People, and UN specialized agencies were asked to convene with governments and indigenous peoples to consider how they could contribute to the success of the Decade of Indigenous People, which officially commenced in December of 1994. In response, at the Forty-seventh World Health Assembly, the World Health Organization (WHO) established a core advisory group comprised of indigenous representatives with special knowledge of the health needs and resources of their communities, thus beginning a long-term commitment to investigate and improve the health of indigenous peoples, which constitutes a global health issue.

The WHO observed that "statistical data on the health status of indigenous peoples [was] scarce. This [was] especially notable for indigenous peoples in Africa, Asia, and Eastern Europe." Nevertheless, snapshots from various countries where such statistics are available show that, in advanced and developing countries alike, indigenous peoples' health status is worse than that of the general population: they suffer from a higher incidence of diabetes in some regions of Australia; higher prevalence of poor sanitation and lack of safe water among Twa households in Rwanda; and a higher rate of childbirths without prenatal care among ethnic minorities in Vietnam. Suicide rates among Inuit youth in Canada are 11 times higher than the national average, and infant mortality rates are higher for indigenous peoples everywhere (Carpenter and McMurchy-Pilkington 2008).

Native Americans cope with significant mental health factors, including depression (Stiffman et al. 2007), suicidal tendencies (Shaughnessy et al. 2004), low self-esteem (Riede 2001), and alienation (Huff 1997). As Herring (1994) indicates, among all the racial/ethnic youth populations in the United States, none seems to be more at risk than Native Americans. Numerous studies have reported higher rates, earlier onset, and more severe consequences of drug abuse among Native American youth compared to their non-Native peers (Schinke et al. 2000; Moncher et al. 1990). The consequences of this abuse among Native American youth are severe: Moncher et al. (1990) found the rate of drug and alcohol abuse by these youths to be associated with delinquency, unemployment, violent behavior, academic failure, and elevated rates of school dropout.

Is the situation getting better or worse? Although the evidence is sparse, there is a disturbing trend of disadvantage across all the health indicators of indigenous peoples. Addressing the indigenous health crisis calls for a holistic vision of health research and the promotion of health interventions that are more future oriented, more integrated, and more pluralistic than at present.

1.1.2   Elevated School Dropout Rates

Education is one of the primary agents of transformation and development. It is an activity, a series of activities, or a process which improves the immediate social, economic, political, human, cultural, or environmental living conditions, and increases the chances of survival of future generations. Education is also a critical factor in human resource development and is essential for a country's economic growth. While the major indicators of socioeconomic development, such as rates of economic growth birth, death, infant mortality, and literacy are all interconnected, the literacy rate has been shown to be the major determinant in the fluctuation of other indicators. There is ample evidence that a high literacy rate, especially in the case of women, correlates with low birth and infant mortality rates, and greater life expectancy. Recognition of this fact has illuminated the need to focus on literacy and elementary education programs, not merely as part of the quest for social justice, but also as a means to foster economic growth, social well-being, and social stability.

The high incidence of school dropouts among indigenous communities is one of the main reasons that these communities lag behind in education (Gautam 2003). One example that demonstrates this is a survey conducted in India by various agencies and compiled by Jharkand Education Project Council (JEPC). Encompassing 25,703 school dropouts in the age group of 6–14 years, the survey reported that compulsion to earn a livelihood forces hundreds of students to leave schools. According to the survey (Indo-Asian News Service, 2007), 26.39 % of students leave school as they are compelled to earn, 25.44 % are engaged in household work, 12.25 % lack interest in studies, and 8 % drop out due to sociocultural reasons. Similarly, an alarmingly high incidence of school dropout was found among Native American and Alaska Native students. This is not a new phenomenon, but one that has persisted throughout the twentieth and early twenty-first centuries (Freeman and Fox 2005). Findings indicate that the number of Native Americans and Alaska

Natives who graduate continues to be a matter of urgent concern. On average, less than 50 % of Native American students in 12 US states graduate each year (Faircloth and Tippeconnic 2010). Indeed, Native American students have become a matter of academic concern across the United States (House 2003). They are the most under-served population (Powers et al. 2003), have the lowest rates of academic achievement and educational success (Sherman 2002), and the highest dropout rate of all racial/ethnic groups in the United States (Jeffries et al. 2004; Gallagher 2000). There are also examples from other parts of the world. For instance, it is estimated that less than 0.5 % of Batwa have completed secondary education (Lewis 2001, p. 16). In Bolivia, indigenous children receive about 3 years less schooling than non-indigenous children (Partridge et al. 1996).

The examples given here are from countries in which data on this issue are available. In other countries, due to a variety of reasons, data on dropout rates are either partial or missing. Lack of accurate data may be due in part to the high mobility of a given population, undercounting of the population, or distrust among this population regarding the use of data by the federal government. The geographic dispersion of Native Americans and Alaska native students, for instance, makes it difficult to collect and report data accurately. Due to such questions regarding the quality of some data sets, many researchers have opted to avoid including data in their reports.

Nevertheless, there is a great need to understand the context and background of education systems in the indigenous communities. Therefore, I wish to present the most frequent reasons for dropping out of school in indigenous communities. First among these is poverty. Poor socioeconomic conditions (poverty) are a major constraint to educational access, making it impossible for marginalized households to invest in education and the related expenses, such as school fees, textbooks, uniforms, meals, and transportation. Children from poor families contribute to family income either directly by working as labor, or indirectly by contributing in doing household chores. Indeed, loss of income is a frequently cited reason for keeping children out of school (Larsen 2003). A survey conducted by the Instituto Nacional Indigenista (INI) indicated that 42,000 indigenous children had dropped out of school mainly because they lacked the financial means to continue studying (Larsen 2003). Honduran school children in rural areas spend an average of 2.9 years in education, while those in urban areas spend and 5.8 years (Lopez 2007). In Oaxaca, Mexico, only 5.2 % of the indigenous population enrolls in middle school or high school, compared to a national average of 26 %, and no more than 2 % of the indigenous population in Oaxaca undertakes occupational studies, compared to a national average of 10.8 % (International Youth Foundation 2000).

Another reason for dropping out of school is the geographical location of the schools and the lack of transport facilities: some remote areas either have no schools at all or if there are any, they are often inaccessible due to poorly maintained roads and lack of public transportation. Some indigenous tribes live in hills or in dense forests with difficult terrain; consequently, geographical isolation and/or lack of infrastructure makes it difficult for public transport services to reach them. It is a challenge to provide education and set up schools and institutions in small, scattered tribal communities situated in remote rural locations.

Discrimination against indigenous children continues to be an issue in education systems and practices (UNESCO 1999) and constitutes yet another cause of high dropout rates. Discrimination can be experienced through the absence of peer relationships, leading to a sense of complete alienation among indigenous children. As a result of a combination of these factors, students from indigenous communities face a series of obstacles on their path to education, including a long commute to school in harsh environmental conditions; poor quality of relationships and occasionally discrimination on the part of teachers and fellow students from nontribal backgrounds; and an inherent disadvantage when negotiating a space for themselves, which they have been denied historically. Psychologically, this has a strong negative impact on children, which again contributes to their dropping out of school (Kumar 2008).

Difficulty in comprehending the language of instruction constitutes yet another obstacle, and another reason behind high dropout rates. Due to language constraints, most indigenous children do not understand the textbooks, which are generally in the regional language. Similarly, nontribal teachers in tribal children's schools do not know the children's native language. Research in child development and pedagogy has indicated that children learn concepts better if these are embedded in contexts that are local, familiar, and consequently meaningful.

One attempt to cope with the language issue was undertaken in the Janshala Program, a collaborative effort of the Government of India and five UN agencies (UNDP, UNICEF, UNESCO, ILO, and UNFPA) to provide programmed support to the ongoing efforts towards achieving Universal Elementary Education. Subsequent evaluation research found that at least at the primary level, students should be taught in their native language. Increasing efforts are being made to deal with these challenges, some of which have been proven by research to be successful. For example, the first 10 years of schooling of the Sami in Norway are conducted in their indigenous language, while in Sweden and Finland, the native language is offered as a medium of instruction only during the first 6 years of school (Lund 2000, p. 10). In other places, a successful way of coping with this challenge is to teach both languages at the same time. Thus, in Guatemala, USAID-funded research has shown that girls in one bilingual education program had higher sixth-grade completion rates than girls in rural schools that did not feature a bilingual curriculum (USAID 1997). Similarly, bilingual education initiatives are key activities of newly formed indigenous organizations in Asia and Africa.

Another factor that affects dropout trends is the rate of literacy within the indigenous community. At a virtually global scale, literacy rates among indigenous and tribal communities are lower than the national average. For example, according to 1991 figures, the literacy rate among tribal peoples in India was only 29.6 %, compared to a national rate of 52 % (Erni and Luithi 2001). Female literacy is considered a significant indicator of educational development within any social group. In Jharkhand State in India, there are 32 different tribal communities, which constitute 26.3 % (6.6 million) of the total population of the State. The average literacy rate in Jharkhand State is 54.13 %, but among some tribes and particularly among women, the literacy rate is as low as 10 % (Kumar 2008).

At the institutional level, research indicates that there are a number of school-related factors associated with higher student dropout rates. Factors that are particularly critical for indigenous students include uncaring teachers; passive teaching methods; irrelevant curricula; inappropriate testing and emphasis on standardized testing, which in some countries leads to built-in failure, due to the way the tests are designed; and the size of the school (especially those with more than a thousand students), which makes it difficult for professionals to be warm, supportive, and caring.

Another reason for the high dropout rates among indigenous communities may be due to a conflict between the education provided at school and the education provided by the community. For many indigenous peoples, traditional education typically includes learning traditional occupations (ILO 2001). For instance, Fuchs and Havighurst (1972) reported that "many Indian children live in homes and communities where the cultural expectations are different and discontinuous from the expectations held by schoolteachers and school authorities" (p. 299). Traditional forms of education include engagement in customary livelihoods, in fields and forests or at sea, with parents and community members. The basic skills transmitted allow children to grow up and survive in often harsh environments. Practical competencies related to these livelihoods are viewed as a necessity for proper socialization. Indeed, prohibiting access to traditional forms of education, by forcing children to participate in non-adapted schooling, may ultimately threaten the children's ability to survive and make a living later on as adults. It may also provoke intergenerational conflict, particularly as educational services often include built-in discriminatory practices.

Figure 1.2 presents a summary of the various reasons for high dropout rates among indigenous children.

Another aspect needs to be highlighted at this point: the dropout problem is actually propelled by a reciprocal process. Many educational institutions and practices are rejecting indigenous peoples, their cultural identities, and their practices (D'Emilio 2001), which in turn causes indigenous communities, comprising both parents and children, to resist the educational services. The rejection of indigenous concerns undermines the necessity and validity of both indigenous knowledge transfer and the traditional forms of education, and thus ultimately rejects the relevance of traditional livelihoods and the indigenous way of life. As Kratli notes,

> school experience is seen as providing the opposite of education: children not only fail to learn how to secure a livelihood, but lose what they were taught in early life and absorb alien and negative values and lifestyles. At school, they are softened, humiliated, trained into dependency, laziness, irresponsibility, lack of discipline and self-esteem. On the other hand, they are made to believe that their school experience raises their social status amongst non-schooled people, so that once back in their communities they often become arrogant, presumptuous and disrespectful (Kratli 2001, p. 38).

Therefore, the issue of dropout prevention must be dealt with holistically. It is imperative to address the reasons that cause these children to drop out, and respond with solutions that are based in the communities' familial, social, and cultural contexts.

There are clear indications that education-support programs need to build on the strengths of the indigenous community, value its culture and history, and at the same

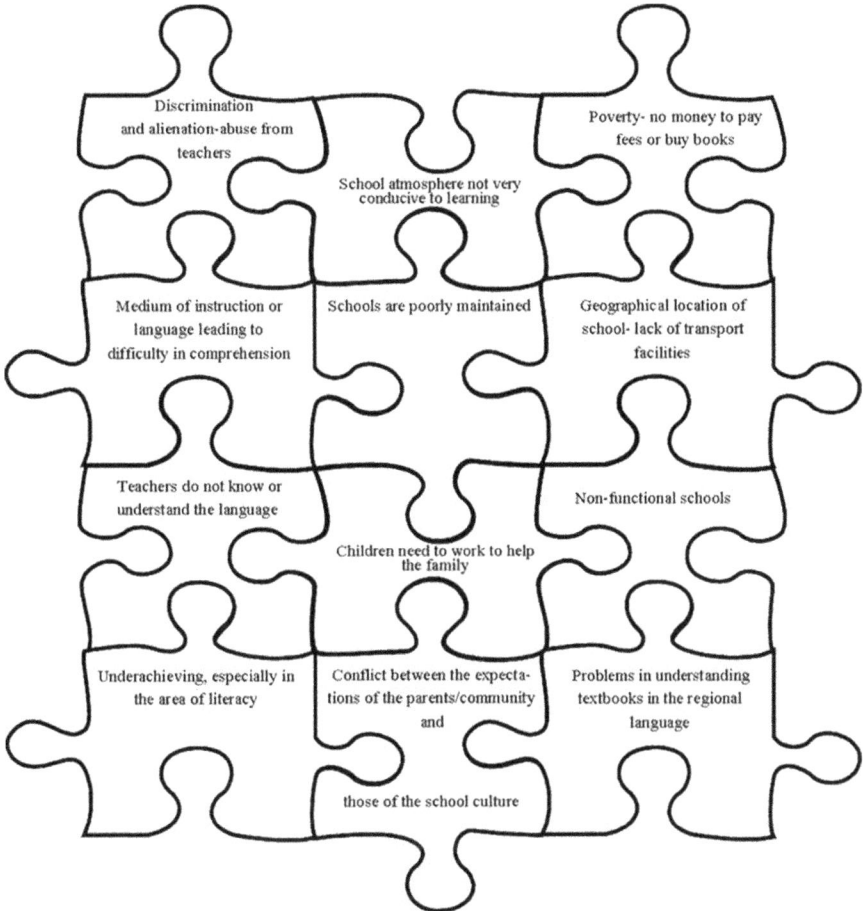

Fig. 1.2 Reasons for school dropout in indigenous communities

time enable a more-or-less seamless integration into mainstream education systems. It is important to examine countries and programs that have dealt with this issue successfully. One way to do this is by conducting comprehensive case studies in states such as Oklahoma (in the United States), where Native American and Alaskan indigenous students appear to be graduating in higher numbers and achieving at higher levels academically compared to their indigenous peers elsewhere in the United States (Moran et al. 2008).

As noted, there is a critical need for a more holistic approach that would move indigenous education beyond the language agenda. Such an approach would involve indigenous education breaking through the cultural domination of national education authorities, by empowering communities to strengthen, implement, and control their own visions of educational programs and practices. The literature includes several successful examples that have led to a decrease in the dropout rates in indigenous communities. Thus, for instance, Brandt (1992) and Bagai and Nundy (2009) have presented recommendations for dealing effectively with dropout rates, and Helme and Lamb (2011) offer examples of what works and what doesn't. To summarize, the description presented herein clarifies and illuminates several important points:

- The lack of accurate reporting of graduation and dropout rates for indigenous students continues to be an issue of concern. The creation of uniform means of calculating and reporting graduation and dropout rates is an important step in illustrating the extent and magnitude of the crisis.
- Issues of education among indigenous children cannot be viewed in isolation from the wider context of structural challenges faced by indigenous peoples as a whole. These challenges involve several socioeconomic and cultural aspects that characterize indigenous communities, children, adults, and households, and distinguish them from the general non-indigenous population. Awareness of particular forms of social exclusion needs to remain at the forefront of problem analysis and solution building.

Up to this point, we have dealt with children who actually attend school. Yet, many children in indigenous communities do not attend school at all; further research is required in order to address this population of children. One recognized reason for nonattendance is child labor.

1.1.3 Child Labor

According to recent global estimates, 211 million children between ages 5–14 are economically active. Of these, approximately 186 million are engaged in child labor. If we include children and youths between the ages of 15–17, the number of child laborers reaches 246 million.

There is evidence suggesting that among indigenous peoples in certain countries there are high numbers of the worst form of child labor. Child labor among indigenous children in South Asia, Southeast Asia, and Latin America takes many forms, including debt-bondage, as found among hill tribe children in Thailand, Central America, and Mexico, and child trafficking, found in Southeast Asia. In Latin America, it is estimated that indigenous children are twice as likely to work as their peers. In Ecuador, nine out of ten indigenous children work, compared to one out of three non-indigenous children (Salazar 1998, p. 6). In Latin America, rural agricultural child labor is mainly found among the indigenous peoples of Mexico, Central America, and the Andean Region, where most indigenous peoples are peasant farmers or wage laborers. For example, it is estimated that more than 50 % of the indigenous agricultural community in Guatemala, Mexico, and Peru survive only as wage laborers. Rural child laborers are involved in sugar cane plantations and rice and coffee harvesting, with studies indicating that indigenous children are employed for more than 40 h per week (Carrasco 1999). In rural areas in Mexico, it is estimated that around 170,000 indigenous children aged 6–14 work for little—if any—wages for their parents, family, or neighbors. In Latin America, indigenous children have been found to work in mines, in Colombia, Peru, and Bolivia (Martinez 2000).

Indigenous values regarding child development and maturing may involve work. IPEC and INDISCO Philippines research has shown that parents in one indigenous community did not necessarily consider child labor to be a problem (Palma-Sealza and Sealza 2000). In the Cordillera region of the Philippines, another research team found that while over 80 % of the children surveyed were involved in some form of child labor, this was rarely considered hazardous or disadvantageous. The attitude among parents was that "children must learn how to work, earn money, contribute to the family's needs, be responsible for one's upkeep and the like" (Reyes-Boquiren 2001, p. 26).

There are clear indications that a growing number of indigenous children are migrating, alone or with their parents, to cities, in search of employment or better opportunities. In India, for example, there has been some documentation of indigenous girls migrating to urban areas to seek employment as domestic workers (Larsen 2003). In Asia, a recent ILO study of socioeconomic vulnerability of indigenous migrants in the cities of Chiang Mai and Chiang Rai in Thailand showed that the majority of street children under the age of 15 were from hill areas in Thailand and Burma, and most were boys who earned a living from selling flowers, begging, or offering sex services (Budaeng et al. 2001). Similar evidence is emerging from other Asian cities either within or neighboring on indigenous areas. In Africa, urban migration of indigenous children and youth is also a growing concern. Indigenous organizations have highlighted the downward spiral of unemployment, delinquency, alcohol and drug addiction, prostitution, and AIDS associated with indigenous children's urban migration (Martinez 2000).

Data on this issue are incomplete, since in some countries the situation is not well documented; overall, data remain relatively weak and sporadic (Larsen 2003). However, as Larsen states, in certain countries, indigenous and tribal children comprise a large portion of urban migrants; hence, this issue demands immediate international attention (Larsen 2003). A comprehensive approach is required, one which can operate on many levels, including international, national, provincial, and community, targeting individuals and families.

1.1.4 The Need for More Extensive Support Services

Many indigenous communities around the world either lack support services, or the existing ones fail to provide adequate responses. Also, indigenous peoples often live in remote areas where they are easily overlooked. Sometimes support services do exist, but the high level of poverty in the indigenous community makes it impossible to pay for treatment or medications. In other places the sparse support services that do exist are situated in distant locations that render them virtually inaccessible, as is the case in El Salvador, for example, regarding both basic services (Lopez 2007) and health services (Larsen 2003). From Central Africa to South and Southeast

Asia, the status of indigenous peoples who have not been granted official citizenship poses serious obstacles to accessing government funded services such as health facilities (Budaeng et al. 2001). As a result of insufficient support services and the absence of accessible healthcare facilities, mortality rates in these communities are higher than the national averages.

The health of the San of Southern Africa was found to be closely linked to marginalization and poverty. Some of the major health problems experienced by the San/Basarwa in Botswana include alcoholism, tuberculosis, and HIV/AIDS. Alcoholism is considered a symptom of marginalization and despondency, as well as a cause of poor health. In addition, many people drink alcohol to deal with hunger (Report of the African Commissions 2005). Also the Batwa in Rwanda, Burundi, and Uganda are severely discriminated in terms of healthcare, due to poverty and marginalization. As a result of their very limited access to primary healthcare, the majority of both adults and children are forced to do without (Report of the African Commissions 2005, p. 52). They are prone to health problems related to diet and nutrition, and Batwa children suffer from chronic malnutrition. Also they do not have access to clean drinking water, since they live in remote areas. Given the lack of money for medicines, compounded with the discrimination they face, the Batwa simply do not go to healthcare centers, and they are left to hope that they will be spontaneously cured of their illnesses, or they practice self-medication. Many Batwa, especially children under 5 years of age, die from malaria, as their families cannot afford the necessary treatment. Child vaccination rates among this community are very low, and at the same time they are exposed to the most dangerous diseases (tetanus, whooping cough, measles, polio). Expecting mothers do not seek prenatal care, they do not take the necessary vaccinations, and they generally give birth at home under non-hygienic conditions. Consequently, many Batwa mothers and children die during childbirth (Report of the African Commissions 2005, p. 54). Another example, based on the results of fieldwork, suggests that the Pygmies do not have access to primary healthcare and mainly rely on traditional medicine. As a result, their communities are affected by many diseases, especially tropical parasitosis, tuberculosis, infectious diseases, respiratory diseases, and infantile infectious diseases, more so than other population groups in their region (Hall and Patrinos 2010). As noted, there is a link between absence, partial, and inadequate support services and limited economic resources and poverty.

1.1.5 Lack of Financial Resources: Poverty

It is widely believed, and in some cases amply documented, that indigenous peoples are the poorest of the poor in terms of income, and that over time this situation has remained constant (Hall and Patrinos 2010). In other words, there is a systematic link between being indigenous and being poor (Word Bank 2005, p. 171). This is true for example in El Salvador and Guatemala, where indigenous peoples mostly live in rural communities (Mullick 2002), as well as in Latin America, South and

Southeast Asia, where indigenous peoples constitute a growing proportion of the new urban migrants, i.e., the urban poor.

This repeated finding prompts the question of causality: what causes indigenous people to be significantly poorer on average than the rest of the population? According to Lumsden (2008), a review of the literature yields six principal (and inter-related) possible explanations for the causes of extreme poverty and disadvantage among indigenous peoples:

1. Spatial disadvantage: geographic characteristics such as climate, vegetation, access to basic infrastructure, and remoteness explain poverty differentials. In China, for example, minorities are twice as likely to live in isolated, remote villages with difficult topography and poor infrastructure.
2. Human capital theory: the lack of education and poor health lead to limited productivity in the labor market, which is one of the major determinants of low income and poverty.
3. Asset-based explanations and poverty traps: in addition to the issue of assets related to human capital, indigenous communities fail to reach even a minimum asset threshold. One result is that they are economically vulnerable, that is, they are unable to cope with events that interfere with routine or undermine stability, which in turn means they cannot escape the condition of poverty.
4. Social exclusion and discrimination: even with a sufficient asset base, the lack of social capital and the ongoing discrimination prohibit access to key "networks" and, thus, increases market segmentation, which effectively means low returns on assets and/or limited access to services and credit, such that the poor remain chronically poor.
5. Cultural and behavioral characteristics: group-level influences and peer effects help inculcate maladaptive, constraining behaviors, such as a "cultural of poverty" and self-reinforcement of stereotypes and stigmas.
6. Dependence on the existing institutional path: in addition to the characteristics and behaviors of the poor, inequality is structurally reproduced via historically determined social and political relationships, exploitation, and "opportunity hoarding" among elites.

In sum, the evidence that can be pieced together so far suggests that there is a systematic link between being indigenous and being poor. Nevertheless, some countries have succeeded in improving the economic conditions of their indigenous communities. Examples include the Hui and Manchu in China, the Aymara in Peru, and to some extent, indigenous communities in India and Vietnam. Currently, the related research priority is to gain a better understanding how these successes came about.

1.1.6   Subjection to Acts of Dispossession and Spirit-Breaking

Studies that investigate the conditions of indigenous nations and the public policies that affect them indicate that these polices share a common denominator: they feature political subjugation, legal and social discrimination, neglect, isolation, and exclusion. Notwithstanding, in the 1960s, the first efforts were made to instigate a political, cultural, legal, and economic revival of these peoples. Currently, with the development of a postcolonial corrective discourse, there is growing recognition of their existence, as well as their status as the largest social sector with a low breaking point. The economic, familial, cultural, and political situation of indigenous nations is the worst among all nations in the world, as was reported by the World Bank in the 1990s: the living conditions of indigenous people are abysmal, and their state of poverty is persistent and severe, especially when compared to those of the non-indigenous population (Psacharopoulos 1994, pp. 206–207).

Certain indigenous societies survive even though they may no longer inhabit their "traditional" lands, owing to migration, relocation, forced resettlement, or having been supplanted by other cultural groups. In many other respects, the transformation of culture of indigenous groups is ongoing, and includes permanent loss of language, loss of lands, encroachment on traditional territories, and disruption of traditional ways of life, due to contamination and pollution of waters and lands. Characteristics common across many indigenous groups include present or historical reliance upon subsistence-based production (based on pastoral, horticultural, and/or hunting and gathering techniques), and a predominantly non-urbanized society.

Since the 29th Ordinary Session of the African Commission on Human and Peoples' Rights (ACHPR) in Libya, in 2001, representatives of the indigenous communities have given strong testimony to their desperate situation and the gross human rights violations of which they are victims. They have informed the ACHPR about the discrimination and contempt they experience, about the dispossession of their lands, the destruction of their livelihood, culture, and identity, and about their lack of access to and participation in political decision making (ACHPR 2005), all of which lead to the dispossession and spirit-breaking of indigenous peoples. They have requested the right to survive as peoples and to have a say in their own future, based on their own culture, languages, identity, hopes, and visions.

The most researched aspect of this issue is language. Thus, for example, for many Māori the alienation from mainstream society is compounded by the loss of a positive identity, which is symbolized by loss of language and self-esteem (Carpenter and McMurchy-Pilkington 2008). Despite a recent renaissance in the isolated pockets where Māori language is in common use, the population is dwindling and the language is in danger of becoming extinct. The journey of Māori culture and language to this state of tentative existence is similar to that of many other colonized and indigenous peoples worldwide. Many indigenous communities around the world are losing their language, if it has not been lost yet. For instance, indigenous languages in El Salvador, with the exception of Nahuatl, have largely disappeared (Lopez 2007).

A major issue in terms of democratic participation and citizenship rights—and one that is closely linked to language issues—is the extent to which indigenous languages are used in administrative and day-to-day matters. In some countries, such as Norway and Finland, indigenous languages are recognized as official languages in certain municipalities, providing people with the right to obtain public services in their own language. In other countries, this may be the case informally, in areas where indigenous peoples form the majority. In most cases, high rates of illiteracy in national languages prevent effective use of public services.

The common characteristics of most indigenous communities, part of which have been presented in this section, have led to the addition of a major clause to the 2007 Declaration on the Rights of Indigenous Peoples. The addendum suggests recognizing the right of indigenous peoples to autonomy, internal self-determination, preservation of their cultural heritage and cultural property, including territory, education, language, and the right to sustain and develop indigenous social and economic systems (Castellino and Gilbert 2003).

Some countries, aware of the difficulties and challenges that indigenous peoples face, have attempted to cope with these issues; thus, there are some positive examples of political recognition and participation, which may be of inspiration. Particularly in regard to the issue of language, several efforts are underway. In Guatemala, for instance, the official language is Spanish, but 23 spoken indigenous languages also exist in the state, an arrangement which permits each indigenous group to use its own language. This practice stands in contrast to that of other countries, which forbid the use of indigenous languages and attempt to eradicate them. Section 6(2) of the South African Constitution of Rights of Communities refers to the need to protect and promote indigenous languages, mentioning the Khoe, San, and Nama languages. In this regard, an important step forward taken in recent years was the approval of a law that sanctions the recognition, respect, promotion, development, and utilization of indigenous languages (Lopez 2007, p. 8). Efforts to preserve the language and culture of indigenous groups are underway in other countries as well, including New Zealand (Carpenter and McMurchy-Pilkington 2008) and Morocco, where on July 31, 2001, King Mohammed VI declared the creation of the Royal Institute for Amazigh Culture and Language.

In conclusion, an important insight that emerges from the—albeit partial—picture presented in this section is that while the severity of the experience of indigenous peoples may differ from country to country, their situation is cause for serious concern and requires intervention. No longer can we sit back and wait for change to happen, and research alone is not enough. Policymakers and practitioners must act immediately at all levels: federal, state, district, local, and tribal.

1.2 Indigenous Communities and Children with Disabilities in the World

The aim of this section is to examine the shared and unique characteristics of indigenous communities vis-à-vis children with disabilities. The main issues brought to the discussion are the state of poor documentation of children with disabilities in indigenous communities, high rates of children with disabilities in indigenous communities, and the absence of—any or adequate—support services.

1.2.1 Disability

Disability is a key concept in this book and, in fact, the manner in which the term is used here also determines the type of data and information sought and the way that information is interpreted. *Children with disabilities* are defined as those whose needs cannot be met within a regular setting, home or family, without extra support. Their needs may stem from a cognitive or intellectual, visual or auditory, physical, motor, communication, behavior and/or emotional disability, or a co morbidity of these. The severity of the disability relates to how much support services the children need. People with a profound or severe limitation need assistance with at least one core activity, such as walking, toileting, dressing, or communicating. In the theoretical and research literature there is a lively discussion regarding the conceptualization, definition, and classification of children with disabilities. There is a direct link between these three components, as represented in the following schematic diagram:

Conceptualization → definition → classification

1.2.1.1 Conceptualization

I shall begin with the subject of conceptualization as it is the first in the schematic order. Although most indigenous communities have experience with disabilities, in some indigenous communities the language does not contain a single word or concept for various disabilities. Likewise, there may be no negative terminology or slang used to refer to disability. For example, among the Navajos there is no word for mental retardation (Joe 1997).

In different places in the world, a single type of disability is designated by different names. Thus, for instance, the expression "intellectual disability," the term selected for use in this manuscript to describe the population of interest, is synonymous with "learning disability," with the North American term "mental retardation," and with the first two parts of the definition of "mental impairment" under the 1983 Mental Health Act (Department of Health and Welsh Office 1982). Here it refers to intellectual disability.

Similarly, a variety of terms are used in different countries to describe children with special needs. In this book, the term of choice is *disability*, since it encompasses a global view of the phenomenon.

In the past 20 years, the concept of disability has evolved, from a medical model that focused on the individual's impairment, to a social model based on functioning and participation, a model that focuses on the external obstacles that limit the individual's range of activities and social participation. We have seen a shift in terminology and an increasing tendency towards viewing disability as a complex process, involving a number of different elements at the individual and societal level. Viewed from this perspective, which populations does the term "children with disabilities" include? Children with disabilities are a diverse and heterogeneous group. Childhood disabilities can affect one or more functional domains, including: cognition, movement, consciousness, language, speech, vision, hearing, and behavior. The term

Table 1.1 Major categories of child disabilities and selected examples

Major categories	Selected examples
Cognitive/Intellectual	Mental retardation/intellectual disability
	Learning disabilities
	Developmental disabilities
Vision and hearing	Blindness and impaired vision
	Deafness and impaired hearing
Physical/Motor	Cerebral palsy
	Paralysis (post-polio, spinal cord or traumatic injury)
Communication	Autism
	The entire spectrum
Behavior	Conduct disorders
	Attention deficit hyperactivity disorder (ADHD)
Emotional	Mood disorder, mental disorder, anxiety

"children with disabilities" is used broadly in this book to refer to disabilities that occur in any of these domains. Table 1.1 below presents several major categories of childhood disabilities and selected examples of disabilities within each category.

1.2.1.2 Classifying the Degree of the Disability

Based on studies conducted in Western countries that have a methodical and structured system for evaluating children with disabilities and maintain databases on this subject, each disability is described in terms of a continuum or a spectrum, ranging from mild to complex. For instance, mental retardation is often classified as mild, moderate, or profound. Defining the child's disability on a continuum raises the issue of the classification of children with disabilities. To identify any particular individual as falling within one of these disability classifications requires the use of a predefined measure. Table 1.2 provides a summary of the different classification methods used, as applied to intellectual disability, by way of example.

As the multiplicity of classification methods demonstrates, disability is a complex, multidimensional experience; consequently, it poses several challenges for the establishment of classification measures. Approaches to measuring and classifying disability vary across countries and thus influence the results. Operational measures of disability vary according to the purpose and application of the data, the conception of disability, the aspects of disability examined (impairments, activity limitations, participation restrictions, related health conditions, environmental factors), the way in which the term is defined and phrased, reporting sources, data collection methods, and expectations of functioning.

As this chapter views disabilities of children in indigenous communities from a global perspective, it is important to use a classification method that can accommodate both the global and local contexts of the indigenous communities. For the conceptual framework of this book, the International Classification of Functioning, Disability and Health (ICF) classification method was adopted, due to several advantages it has over other classification systems.

Table 1.2 Summary-example of the different methods used in the classification of intellectual disabilities

Classification of intellectual disabilities	Focus
DSM — Diagnostic and Statistical Manual of Mental Disorders (American Psychological Association)	Presents a definition and rules for determining levels of intellectual disabilities, but is used primarily for classifying a wide range of "psychic" disabilities, some of which are related to intellectual disabilities
ICD — The International Classification of Functioning, Disability and Health	Includes rules for determining various levels of intellectual disabilities and is known as an internationally accepted method of identifying illnesses and physical states, including those that can be attributed to intellectual disabilities
ICF — International Classification of Functioning, Disability and Health (WHO — World Health Organization)	This method classifies functioning in terms of structure and functioning of the body, in addition to activities, participation, and contextual factors
AAMR — American Association on Mental Retardation	The AAMR has taken significant steps away from a clinically oriented perspective towards a multidimensional approach in defining intellectual disabilities. The AAMR definition gives more credence to the "state" of interaction between the individual and the social environment. Such descriptions of severity are considered to be more functional, relevant, and oriented to service delivery and outcomes than the labeling classification

The first such advantage is that this method allows us to understand functioning and disability as a dynamic interaction between environmental conditions (including community, family, and parents) and contextual factors. According to the ICF, disability is recognized when an individual's ability to perform daily activities, carry out social roles, and/or participate in typical communal activities is impaired. According to this classification system, understanding disability means taking into account both the individual and the social consequences of the impairment. The focus is on the interaction between the individual's physical and personal characteristics and the *environment* in the broadest sense of the word, encompassing the individual's social, cultural, and physical world. Thus, in order to understand disability it is necessary to focus not only on the individual but also on the family and/or the social group with whom the individual coexists, and to examine the ways in which the individual, family, and society function and cope with the consequences of the disability within their particular social and cultural milieu. Within the ICF's classification system of functioning, both the individual and the environment are in focus. The ICF classification system is designed to be culturally neutral and applicable in cross-cultural frameworks. The personal, practical, and social consequences of impairment will differ depending on factors such as gender, economic and social class, culture, caste, and geographical remoteness. Different kinds of impairments are understood differently and will have different consequences in different cultures.

Another advantage of the ICF is the fact that it was developed over a long process, in which academics, clinicians, and — importantly — persons with disabilities were involved. Moreover, the ICF classification system can be used to understand

and measure the positive aspects of functioning, such as bodily functions, activities, participation, and environmental facilitation. The ICF also contains a classification of environmental factors, perceived as either facilitators or barriers, which is used to describe the world in which people with different levels of functioning must live and act. The ICF further distinguishes between a person's capacities to perform actions and the actual performance of those actions in real life, a subtle difference that helps illuminate the effect of the environment and can serve to demonstrate ways in which modifying the environment can help improve performance.

A final advantage, which is especially important for anyone dealing with children with disabilities in a global context, is that the ICF is universal because it covers all human functioning and treats disability as a continuum, rather than as a means for categorizing people. Furthermore, disability according to the ICF is considered a matter of degree, that is, more or less, not yes or no. The ICF serves a range of purposes, such as research, surveillance, and reporting, in which it is used to describe and measure the degree of disability. It can also be applied and used by support services, for example, for assessing individual functioning, goal setting, treatment, and monitoring; measuring outcomes and evaluating services; determining eligibility for welfare benefits; and developing health and disability surveys.

Clearly, relying on a stable definition or classification system that allows for comparison over time and place has critical implications for epidemiological research. Taxonomy in this field is particularly difficult because professionals and consumers come from a range of backgrounds and have different purposes, such as advocacy, education, medical care, and service provision. Consequently, it would be even more effective to have a conceptual framework that could map the various definitions and classification systems in a way amenable to scientific investigation and support services. This is important if we want to know the "true prevalence" of children with disabilities in indigenous communities.

As a first step towards establishing such a conceptual framework, I propose using an existing module, namely, the Ten Questions Screen for Child Disability from the Multiple Indicator Cluster Survey (MICS). Twenty-six of the fifty countries that participated in the third round of MICS, administered in 2005–2008, included this optional child disability module. MICS is one of the first surveys to use a single screen for disability across a wide range of countries. By adopting the module from this survey, I hope to raise awareness about the number and the conditions of children with disabilities in indigenous communities. The Ten Questions screen was designed as a tool for both identifying children at increased risk for disability, who in turn are referred for comprehensive clinical evaluations.

1.2.2 Children with Disability: Poor Documentation in the Indigenous Community

Disabilities occur in every nation and community in the world. The first question that research should ask is what is the likely prevalence of children with disabilities in a specific community? In this book, the question pertains to the indigenous community. Although the majority of children in the world live in developing countries and in indigenous communities and therefore may be at high risk for disability, to date, the issue of disability among children in indigenous communities has received only limited attention. Consequently, there is little information available on the prevalence and causes of disability in this group. As Glasson et al. noted, "[c]hild disability among indigenous peoples continues to remain poorly documented and data is generally limited, disparate, and of low quality" (Glasson et al. 2005, p. 627).

There are many reasons for the paucity of population studies focusing on indigenous children with disabilities, most critical among them are cultural diversity, geographical dispersion, and the relatively small size of these populations. There are also major cultural differences between the indigenous peoples of a given country. For example, there are 562 federally recognized Native American tribes in the United States (US Department of the Interior, 2005). These small, culturally distinct populations create sampling problems that make it nearly impossible to draw generalizations about Native Americans as a group. As Native American populations constitute small percentages of the general US population, national-scale studies nearly always relegate them to the category of "other ethnic groups" and usually include only urban Native Americans in the sampling frame. Two additional reasons for the paucity of studies about children with disabilities in indigenous communities around the world are the difficulty of collecting data in settings where few children with disabilities are formally identified and receiving services, and a tendency among researchers and health providers to view childhood disabilities as a low priority in populations where infant and child mortality rates are still in great excess. Yet another possible obstacle to documenting children with disabilities may be that they are concealed by their parents, due to a perception of social stigma or other cultural beliefs and practices. In Nigeria, for instance, certain indigenous communities believe that if a child is born with a mental disability, the family has been cursed by the gods and is being punished for evil doing. In many African indigenous communities, grand mal epilepsy is considered a form of severe mental illness (Omigbodun 2004). Therefore, families are known to manage this stigma by locking up children with mental disabilities and epilepsy, keeping them away from the prying eyes of neighbors. Often this leads the parents to abandon the child, who is thus left to endure slow starvation (Desjarlais et al. 1995). In addition, many of the children in these African communities lack access to healthcare, due to beliefs, poverty, and poor health access (Omigbodun 2008).

Problems exist in gathering data, even when researchers conduct systematic studies. Thus, for example, Glasson et al. (2005) noted that during their investigation (about assessment of intellectual disability among Aboriginal Australians), much of the information on children was found to be either missing, incomplete, or vaguely coded. As the collection of information on the status of indigenous peoples can be a very sensitive issue, certain questions may have been omitted or not recorded electronically.

In a stable population, the prevalence (i.e., the number of existing cases) of a certain illness is a function of its incidence (the number of new cases per unit of time) and the persistence or duration of disease. Although incidence is preferable to prevalence as a measure for investigating risk and etiology, data on the incidence of children with disability in any population are unattainable, due to the absence of longitudinal data from conception, or birth, to death. Thus, the epidemiology of children with disabilities must generally be inferred from prevalence estimates taken at various time points and locations, based on cross-sectional data. These estimates have to be interpreted with caution, as they are indicators of risk confounded by variations in the populations' survival rates. Not unlike the case in low-income countries, the incidence of disability in indigenous communities—though immeasurable—is most likely elevated. This is due not only to increased exposure to the many known causes of brain injury and abnormal development (discussed below under risk factors) but also to the limited medical care and support services available once the exposure has occurred. In countries with well-developed services for children with disabilities, administrative data and registries provide a useful source of population-based data on childhood disabilities; however, in most countries where indigenous communities live, health, education, and rehabilitation services for children with special needs are sparse or not universally available, and children with disabilities are less likely than their peers to attend school (Miles 1997; Durkin et al. 2000; Committee on Nervous System Disorders in Developing Countries 2001).

Another reason for the absence of administrative data is the "key informant" approach, which involves interviewing teachers, healthcare providers, community leaders, and other key persons in the community in order to identify children with disabilities. This approach, too, has been shown to overlook disabilities that are not visible, such as hearing and cognitive disabilities, and to include children from outside the population of interest (Thorburn et al. 1991). An approach that overcomes these limitations is the "two-phase prevalence survey," which involves door-to-door surveys and individualized screening of all the children in the community for disabilities, followed by diagnostic assessments of children who screened positive, and sampling of those who screened negative (Shrout and Newman 1989). This approach provides the most comprehensive coverage in settings with limited services, and for this reason it might be expected to generate higher estimates of prevalence than the alternative approaches. In addition to differences in basic approaches, case-finding methods vary also in terms of inclusion criteria, case definitions, and diagnostic criteria used.

The issue of the assessment of children with disabilities also poses a problem in terms of data collection. Assessment information must include data regarding the type of diagnostic or assessment instrument used for the purpose of classifying the child's disability, particularly since most existing, standard diagnostic and assessment/instruments were developed to target children from majority cultures, and therefore their use with indigenous populations may lead to bias or misdiagnoses.

Due to the lack of assessment, treatment, and services for children with disabilities, many of these children—despite being referred to a range of service systems—end up in the juvenile justice system, "consigned to incarceration rather than treatment" (The Senate Community Affairs References Committee 2005). Given all of these obstacles, it is difficult to provide precise information on the prevalence of children with disabilities in indigenous communities.

All the same, it is important to note that there are a number of countries in the world, such as Australia, where there is a government strategy and a matching framework for conducting systematic documentation and study of indigenous children with disabilities. This enables examination of the contexts and causality of phenomena, and provides interesting data. Thus, an interesting study was conducted in Australia on the relationship between intellectual disability, indigenous status, and risk of repeat offenses by juvenile offenders. The study conducted by the NSW Department of Juvenile Justice (2003) revealed that young people in custody reported symptoms consistent with several conditions: 88 % of the reports coincided with a mild, moderate, or severe psychiatric disorder; 30 % with Attention Deficit Hyperactivity Disorder; and 21 % with schizophrenia; while 10–13 % were assessed as having an intellectual disability. In addition, a later study found that 8 % of young men and 12 % of young women reported having attempted suicide in the previous 12 months; 21 % of young men and 56 % of young women reported alcohol abuse in the hazardous/harmful range; and, 51 % reported problems resulting from drug abuse (NSW Department of Juvenile Justice, 2004–2006). The report also determined the figure of 10 % to be a "culture-fair" estimate of intellectual disability among the Aboriginal and Torres Strait Islander youths in custody (NSW Young People in Custody Health Survey 2003). Data are lacking not only as to the prevalence and extent of this phenomenon but also as to the type/classification of the disabilities. Assessments of prevalence and classification would enable the examination of context and causality.

Notwithstanding the documentation difficulties and the meager amount of data that are available, the picture that does emerge suggests that the number of children with disabilities in indigenous communities is relatively high. However, if appropriate prevention and intervention strategies are to be provided, there is an urgent need for more detailed information on the prevalence and patterns of disabilities among children in indigenous communities. Robust evidence helps to make well-informed decisions about disability policies and programs; consequently, without more specific information on geographical locations, levels of disability, and children profiles, the development and targeting of services and policies addressing the needs of indigenous communities will continue to be a major problem. Robust evidence helps to make well-informed decisions about disability policies and programs. Therefore, acquiring more accurate information regarding the number of people with disabilities as well as their circumstances can facilitate efforts to remove disabling barriers and provide people with disabilities the necessary services to enable them to increase their participation in daily life and social activities.

Diagnosis of a child's disability requires a process of recognition that includes a variety of methods, assessment instruments, and professionals. A framework useful for the purposes of this investigation is presented in Bagnato and Neisworth's (1991) definition of assessment, which depicts assessment as a flexible, collaborative decision-making process, in which teams of parents and professionals work together to identify the needs of children and their families. The assessment practices recommended by The Division for Early Childhood of the Council for Exceptional Children (DEC) (Neisworth and Bagnato 2005) could also be used.

The accuracy of disability screening and assessment tools is subject to debate and scrutiny, particularly with regard to the extent to which these mechanisms are culturally relevant for the indigenous population. Westerman, an indigenous person who runs indigenous psychological services in Western Australia, notes that some attempts have been made to develop assessment tools suitable for indigenous people, but much more work still needs to be done. In developing assessment tools, the focus should be on the known strengths of the indigenous people. For the notion of assessment to be more acceptable to indigenous people, tools need to have "faith validity," that is, they need to make sense to indigenous people, and indigenous people need to be able to relate to them. Those administering the relevant tests also need cultural competence training.

Despite the difficulties, obtaining information that can help identify children with disabilities in indigenous communities is important, as it serves a number of uses. First, it can alert governments to the need to adapt or extend education and other services in order to address the particular needs of these children and their families, in a manner that suits the population's requirements. Second, it will enable international comparisons of prevalence, which may confirm the extent to which the identification of this condition is affected by cultural influences (Fombonne 2009), etiological factors, or a combination of both. To date, studies on cultural indigenous factors and disabilities have received little attention. Third, this type of data can be useful for devising and testing procedures suitable for identifying children with this condition in indigenous cultures, rather than presuming that assessment tools developed in other countries are adequate.

1.2.3 High Rates of Children with Disabilities in the Indigenous Community: Explanatory Factors

The data presented in this section must be viewed with caution, in light of the difficulties presented in the previous section. The sparse data that exist regarding children with disabilities in indigenous communities points to a significantly high prevalence of children with disabilities in some indigenous communities. One example is the high rate of disorders related to substance abuse found among Native American/Alaska Native youths, which represents a significant problem affecting these communities (Beals et al. 1997; Dixon et al. 2007). In a study conducted among indigenous adolescents from the Northern Midwest and Canada, the lifetime conduct disorder rate was found to be more than twice the rate found in the general population (Whitbeck et al. 2008). Also, in a study analyzing data among a sample of Northern Plains adolescents aged 14–16 years and two comparison groups, Native American youths demonstrated higher rates of disruptive behavior disorders, conduct disorder, and oppositional defiant disorder than did either of the comparison samples (Beals et al. 1997). These statistics are important, since behavior and mental health problems experienced during childhood and adolescence may significantly impact growth and development, school performance, and peer and family relationships, as well as lead to an increased risk of suicide (Bhatia and Bhatia 2007). In Australia, the National Aboriginal and Torres Strait Islander Social Survey of 2002 estimated that Indigenous Australians are 1.5 times more likely to have a disability (including physical, mental, and intellectual) than non-Indigenous Australians (Australian Bureau of Statistics 2004). Similarly, Glasson et al. (2005) examined the Disability Services Commission of Western Australia's database of clients since 1953 and found over-representation of intellectual disabilities among indigenous people in Western Australia. Although indigenous people comprise 3.5 % of the population in Western Australia, they represented 7.4 % of all people registered for intellectual disabilities services. The level of intellectual disability was assessed as borderline or mild in 40.7 % of cases, moderate in 19.9 %, and severe or profound in 12.1 %, while levels were not specified in 27.2 % cases. The median life expectancy was 55.1 years for men and 64.9 years for women, yet the mean age at death of 19.6 years. The leading causes of death were respiratory diseases, diseases of circulatory system, and accidents (Glasson et al. 2005). Employing the same database used by Glasson et al. (2005), Leonard et al. (2005) investigated the social correlates of intellectual disabilities of unknown cause in a group of children born between 1983 and 1992 in Western Australia. Children of indigenous women were found to be 2.83 times more likely to have mild to moderate intellectual disabilities and 1.67 times more likely to have severe intellectual disabilities than non-indigenous children. Having an indigenous parent was a significant sociodemographic predictor associated with mild to moderate intellectual disabilities (Frize et al. 2008). The sparse data existing and presented here point to a profusion of children with disabilities in indigenous communities. The question is: what is the reason for this?

Based on the limited data available, this section highlights causes and risk factors that contribute to the prevalence of disabilities in indigenous communities.

Genetic factors—First, there are reasons related to the genetic characteristics of indigenous communities. For example, a number of relatively rare genetic disorders, which pose life-threatening dangers or significant disability among certain Native American and Alaska Native populations, have been observed and reported; some of these are unique conditions, and others demonstrate unusual frequency among certain Native American populations. The examples presented here are disorders that have been the focus of considerable investigation due to their frequent occurrence among Native American communities: severe combined immune deficiency syndrome (Jones et al. 1991), familial Navajo arthropathy (Singleton et al. 1990), congenital adrenal hyperplasia (Hirschfeld and Fleshman 1969), Kuskokwim syndrome (Wright 1970), metachromatic leukodystrophy (Pastor-Soler et al. 1994), and congenital joint contractures resembling arthrogryposis, found in the Inuit people of the Kuskokwim River Delta in Alaska. Another genetics-related factor *induced by certain behaviors is* the phenomenon of consanguineous marriage (typically between first-cousins), which results in increased homozygosity for deleterious mutations. This phenomenon is especially prominent among some populations in South Asia, the Middle East, and North Africa. Consanguinity has been linked to increased prenatal mortality and disabling childhood conditions in a number of populations (World Health Organization 1996; Durkin et al. 2000). Another factor that influences disability and is related to certain behaviors is the introduction of adverse prenatal and perinatal conditions that are known to be risk factors associated for example with intellectual disability. These significant contributors, accounting for some 36 % of cases of intellectual disability according to Glasson et al. (2005), include maternal drug or alcohol use during pregnancy, physical trauma, multiple births, birth complications, infections, and low birth weight. A number of prenatal, postnatal, and childhood infections, including rubella, syphilis and meningitis, among others, can result in damage to the developing nervous system and cause long-term disabilities in children (Committee on Nervous System Disorders in Developing Countries 2001).

Factors related to the physical environment—A child's environment has a huge impact on the experience and extent of disability. Impoverished physical and social environments, landmines, natural and human-induced disasters, lack of road safety, the absence of basic injury prevention strategies, and child abuse and neglect together can either be a direct cause of handicap, or at the very least they leave children in many low-income communities exposed to excess hazards that are likely to increase the risk of developmental disabilities (Richman 1993). The degraded physical environments in which many indigenous communities live constitute an additional factor which increases the risk of contracting general infections (some of which can lead to developmental disability), respiratory diseases, and parasitic diseases. This factor may be especially relevant in remote areas (in Australia, for example) where sanitation is poor and the water supply may be contaminated (Torzillo et al. 1995; Gracey et al. 1997). High-level exposure to certain environmental contaminants such as lead and methylmercury are known to be a direct cause of disabilities (Mendola et al. 2002). Folate deficiency very early in pregnancy is a well-established risk factor for neural tube defects, such as spina bifida, which result in motor disability and in some cases, intellectual impairment among surviving infants.

Factors related to the social environment—It has been established that poor socioeconomic status constitutes a risk factor for disabilities (Durkin 2002). Environments with higher levels of violence and dangerous levels of alcohol consumption in the indigenous community (Helps and Harrison 2004; Chikritzhs and Brady 2006) are likely to lead to higher rates of fetal alcohol syndrome and acquired brain injury in indigenous children (Harris and Bucens 2003). Other Australian data suggest that indigenous mothers to children with intellectual disability tend to be younger and less educated (Australian Bureau of Statistics 2003), to reside in remote rural regions (Gee and O'Neill 2001), and to be less likely to seek early prenatal care (Crowe 1995), all of which can be disadvantageous to childhood development.

Although there is a close linkage between poverty and disability, little research has been carried out analyzing the mechanisms behind this relationship (Elwan 1999). An abundance of literature has shown that in high-income countries, the living conditions among individuals with disabilities are of lower standards than those of non-disabled individuals. While there is less of a focus on this relationship in low-income countries, a few recent studies and reviews have documented the same pattern also in Africa (in particular: Eide and Loeb 2003; Loeb and Eide 2004).

The relationship between disability and poverty is bidirectional (Yeo and Moore 2003), so that disability may increase the risk of poverty, and poverty may increase the risk of disability.

A growing body of empirical evidence from across the world indicates that people with disabilities and their families are more likely to experience economic and social disadvantage than those without disability. Yet information is scant on the dynamics that can explain how the presence of impairments affects the economic and social life of people, or how poverty affects the occurrence of disability in developing countries. Nevertheless, there is sufficient knowledge to conclude that people with disabilities are at risk of being and remaining among the poorest. On an individual level, the relationship depends on the social and economic circumstances under which the individual lives.

Among the poverty-related conditions that can cause disability is children's lack of access to proper nutrition. Protein and energy malnutrition are two of the strongest predictors of poor mental performance (Grantham-McGregor 2002); not surprisingly, children with developmental disabilities are at increased risk for malnutrition, which, in turn, impacts adversely on their survival and ability to benefit from educational interventions. An important recent study from sub-Saharan Africa demonstrated a possible direct association between under nutrition and permanent hearing loss in 0–3 months old infants (Olusanya 2010).

Micronutrient deficiencies, a manifestation of malnutrition, can affect child development both directly and by interacting with infections. Indeed, Micronutrient deficiencies may be the leading cause of developmental disabilities worldwide. Specifically, vitamin A deficiency in childhood, if severe enough to result in exophthalmia, is likely to be the leading cause of childhood blindness in the world. The World Health Organization estimates that it causes 70 % of the estimated half a million new cases of blindness or partial blindness occurring in children each year (World Health Organization 2002). In addition to the direct effects of vitamin A deficiency on the eyes and vision, it further contributes to childhood disability by increasing the risk of contracting measles and other serious childhood infections that can result in long-term disability (Sommer and West 1997). Dietary deficiency of another micronutrient, iodine, is still prevalent in many less-developed countries and has been described as the leading cause of preventable intellectual disabilities in the world (Hetzel 1983). In utero exposure to maternal iodine deficiency during the first two trimesters of pregnancy can damage the developing brain, causing permanent cognitive disability as well as early onset motor, hearing, and speech disabilities. A third micronutrient deficiency, iron deficiency anemia, is also widespread in low-income countries. In some populations, up to 50 % of pregnant women, infants, and children are affected (Viteri 1998). In addition to dietary deficiency, other risk factors for iron deficiency anemia in low-income countries include hookworm and other helminthes infestations, malaria, diarrheal disease, and poverty. Iron deficiency anemia may contribute to the risk of childhood disability by lowering immunity, impairing vitamin A absorption and thyroid hormone transformation, increasing lead absorption, and increasing the risk of low birth weight (Scholl and Hediger 1994).

Poverty is related to disability through lack of necessary healthcare and medication; absence of sanitary installations; contamination of the air, soil, and drinking water; insufficient access to limited resources such as food, clean water, and land; and lack of support for high costs associated with the impairment (Elwan 1999; Yeo and Moore 2003). Moreover, in an impoverished and disadvantaged setting an existing health condition can easily turn into a disability, whether due to an inaccessible environment or insufficient health and rehabilitation services.

One way of addressing the complex issue of high disability rates in indigenous communities is to ensure the presence and proper functioning of multifaceted support services.

1.2.4 Support Services

In this book, the term "support services" refers to the entirety of existing services that address the unique needs of children with disabilities, among them educational, welfare, and medical services, to mention but a few. Most indigenous communities live in the periphery, far away from urban centers; infrastructure such as roads, water, and electricity do not reach these tribal localities. Reduced accessibility and connectivity has further prevented indigenous children with disabilities from improving their lives. Similarly, women living in rural and remote areas may find it difficult to reach a center that can provide prenatal care and neonatal screening; consequently, they use these services only infrequently (Glasson et al. 2005). For example, research refers to a large proportion of documented cases of Aborigines living in non-metropolitan areas, where appropriate services may be difficult to access: 30 % of these cases were recorded as inactive for receipt of services. These findings suggest that either contact with clients from remote areas was lost or that social or cultural barriers were preventing service utilization (Glasson et al. 2005).

In other cases, indigenous communities may have support services within their reach, but there is no professional there who can evaluate and treat children with certain disabilities. One example among many is in the area of mental disabilities: existing health services do not address the mental health needs of the millions of children in these resource-constrained settings. A stark reality that captures the dearth of resources is the statistical finding that there is not even one psychiatrist per 100,000 people in much of South East Asia and the proportion is even smaller — per one million people — in most of sub-Saharan Africa (World Health Organization, 2005). The few child psychiatrists that are available have to participate in all aspects of mental healthcare, leaving little or no time for them to develop services specifically for children (Olatawura 2005). In addition, of the few children who do manage to see a psychiatrist, many are lost to follow-up and very little is known about the outcome of the visits, because the programs that are available are very poorly organized and lack the multidisciplinary teams needed to provide collaborative care (Omigbodun 2004; Dogra and Omigbodun 2004).

In cases with more than one disability or medical condition, children's symptoms were either overlooked or attributed to preexisting conditions or to known medical problems; in the absence of a preexisting condition, the presentation of dual or multiple disabilities complicated the diagnostic process (Bevan-Brown 2004).

Sometimes professionals in support services are forced to use assessment tools, procedures, and resources which are inappropriate, or do not suit the needs of the indigenous community. In Australia, for example, parents expressed their desire for more culturally appropriate assessment measures and procedures and for more Māori services, service providers, and professionals (Bevan-Brown 2004).

In one example of cultural inappropriateness, a Māori child was provided with a computer, which came with word predictive software in English, but no macron software or Māori dictionary (Bevan-Brown 2004). Also the test itself was severely criticized:

> The only thing [the assessor] knew to do was throw a WISC [Wechsler Intelligence Scale for Children] at him, which she did, but she hadn't even modified it for New Zealand conditions, much less Māori kids [or the Māori language] ... I was absolutely horrified—how many stars on the bloody American flag? Like an 11 year old out of kura kaupapa Māori is going to know that! What is the capital of Brazil?—how useful is that! It was just so inappropriate, I mean, Hape knew a lot of the stuff she [was] asked simply because we live in a household where we look at stuff like that, but how many 11 year olds who are in kura kaupapa Māori know who Charles Darwin was—in fact how many 11 year olds in New Zealand know who Charles Darwin was, they don't hit that till high school ... I just couldn't believe the inappropriateness of it (Bevan-Brown 2004, p.22).

The foregoing discussion has cultural implications for the assessment of children with disability who come from different backgrounds. First, the disability screening tools need to be considered. When cultures are very diverse, different assessment methods may have to be used in each. A second consideration is the availability of culturally trained personnel to oversee screening and diagnostic services. Yet another cultural aspect, parental literacy, may affect parents' participation in screening and their engagement in face-to-face interviews; however, obtaining information from parents may constitute an important part of the assessment process, as in the case of identifying autistic disorders.

In addition, more often than not, service providers do not live in the tribal communities of their clients or patients and consequently are not sufficiently familiar with the physical, psychological, and political exigencies that the family experiences on a daily basis. This basic inequity of context can undermine the utility of service provided (Vraniak 1997).

In the absence of support services, it is likely that traditional healers will continue to act as support service providers, until such time as modern services become more accessible. It is no surprise that indigenous people seek help from traditional healers, given that the latter are abundantly available within the communities and, as the large signposts declare, they offer "cure all" services.

It is essential that the process of designing and providing adequate support services to indigenous communities be guided by careful policy development and implementation, as this input will determine the development of key aspects of the system of services. Due attention must be paid to the task of training a greater number of pediatric professionals. It is important to establish partnerships — between professionals working in tertiary centers and those working in secondary and primary care settings.

The support services provided to children in schools are just one phase, which will be described in a separate chapter of this book; however, support systems must be made available for the long term, addressing the needs of individuals throughout their lifespan. It is important to note that certain countries have reported substantial progress on this issue. For instance, the Millennium Development Goals (MDGs), agreed on by the international community in the year 2000, was endorsed by 189 countries. This unified set of development objectives aims to address the needs of the world's poorest and most marginalized people, and the intention is to achieve these goals by 2015. In a similar intent to better address the needs of the Native American communities, the Office of Special Education Programs (OSEP) and the Individuals with Disabilities Education Act of the US Department of Education required the Bureau of Indian Education (BIE) to report annually on 20 performance indicators related to the provision of special education services to children ages 3–21.

Implementation of the important and constructive principles presented here is crucial for devising future plans in the cycle of "prevention — intervention — research," which is–ultimately — the goal of professionals whose work focuses on helping children with disabilities in indigenous communities around the world. While it is clear that using multiple sources and observing possible links between trends constitutes an efficient strategy in this process, the next step may be to establish systems that allow connections to be observed across generations and jurisdictions. Such research processes would have the capacity not only to identify the intergenerational risk factors that impact child disadvantage but also to provide clues on how social policies could be used for intervention purposes. This sort of intersectional collaboration is essential both for understanding the determinants of disabilities as well as for providing the most appropriate and cost-effective services to these children and their families. There are exciting opportunities ahead for making major inroads into this field — opportunities that must not be missed while grappling with the methodological challenges described herein.

References

African Commission on Human and Peoples' Rights. (2005). *Working group of experts on indigenous populations/communities* (Report of the African Commissions). Submitted in accordance with the Resolution on the Rights of Indigenous Populations of Africa. Banjul, The Gambia: ACHPR.

Australian Bureau of Statistics, Australian Institute of Health and Welfare. (2003). *The health and welfare of Australia's Aboriginal and Torres Strait Islander Peoples, 2003, Cat no. 4704.0.* Canberra: ABS.

Australian Bureau of Statistics, Australian Institute of Health and Welfare. (2004). *Year Book Australia, Cat. No. 1301.0.* Canberra: Australian Bureau of Statistics.

Bagai, S., & Nundy, N. (2009). *Tribal education—A fine balance*. Mumbai: Dasra.

Bagnato, S. J., & Neisworth, J. T. (1991). *Assessment for early intervention: Best practices for professionals*. New York: Guilford.

Bank, W. (2005). Cited in International Work Group for Indigenous Affairs (2006). *The Indigenous World, 2006*, 171.

Beals, J., Piasecki, J., Nelson, S., Jones, M., Keane, E., Dauphinais, P., et al. (1997). Psychiatric disorder among American Indian adolescents: Prevalence in Northern Plains youth. *Journal of the American Academy of Child and Adolescent Psychiatry, 36*, 1252–1259.

Bevan-Brown, J. (2004). *Māori perspectives of autistic spectrum disorder: Report to the Ministry of Education*. Wellington, New Zealand: Ministry of Education.

Bhatia, S. K., & Bhatia, S. C. (2007). Childhood and adolescent depression. *American Family Physician, 75*, 73–80.

Brandt, E. A. (1992). The American Indian female dropout. *Journal of American Indian Education, 31*(3), 3–21.

Budaeng, K., Panadda, B., & Prasit, L. (2001). *Study on the socio-economic vulnerability of urban-based tribal peoples in Chiang Mai and Chiang Rai* (Report for the International Labour Office). Chiang Mai, Thailand: Center for Ethnic Studies and Development, Social Research Institute, Chiang Mai University.

Carpenter, V. M., & Mcmurchy-Pilkington, C. (2008). Cross-cultural researching: Maori and Pakeha in Te Whakapakari. *Qualitative Research, 8*(2), 179–196.

Carrasco, D. (1999, 8 December). New efforts to end child labour. *InterPress Third World News Agency*.

Castellino, J., & Gilbert, J. (2003). Self-determination, indigenous peoples and minorities. *Macquarie Law Journal, 3*, 155–178.

Chikritzhs, T., & Brady, M. (2006). Fact or fiction? A critique of the National Aboriginal and Torres Strait Islander social survey 2002. *Drug and Alcohol Review, 25–8*.

Committee on Nervous System Disorders in Developing Countries. (2001). *Neurological, psychiatric and developmental disorders: Meeting the challenge in the developing world*. Washington, DC: Institute of Medicine.

Crow, C. (1995). Cultural issues. *Australian Family Physician, 24*, 1461–1466.

D'Emilio, L. (2001). *Voices and processes towards pluralism: Indigenous education in Bolivia* (New Education Division Documents No. 9). Stockholm: Department for Democracy and Social Development, DESO, SIDA.

Department of Health & Welsh Office. (1982). *Mental Health Act*. London: HMSO.

Desjarlais, R., Eisenberg, L., Good, B., & Kleinman, A. (1995). *World mental health: Problems and priorities in low-income countries*. Oxford: Oxford University Press.

Dixon, A. L., Yabiku, S. T., Okamoto, S. K., Tann, S. S., Marsiglia, F. F., Kulis, B., et al. (2007). The efficacy of a multicultural prevention intervention among urban American Indian youth in the southwest US. *The Journal of Primary Prevention, 28*, 547–568.

Dogra, N., & Omigbodun, O. O. (2004). Learning from low-income countries: What are the lessons? Partnerships in mental health are possible without multidisciplinary teams. *British Medical Journal, 329*, 1184–1185.

Durkin, M. S., Khan, N. Z., & Davidson, L. L. (2000). Prenatal and postnatal risk factors for mental retardation among children in Bangladesh. *American Journal of Epidemiology, 152*, 1024–32.

Durkin, M. (2002). The epidemiology of developmental disabilities in low-income countries. *Mental Retardation and Developmental Disabilities Research Review, 8*(3), 206–211.

Eide, A.H., Loeb, M.E. (2003). *Living conditions among people with activity limitations in Namibia*. A National representative study. (SINTEF Report No. STF 78 A034503). Oslo: SINTEF Unimed.

Elwan, A. (1999). *Poverty and disability: A survey of the literature* (Social protection discussion paper series No. 9932). Washington D.C: the World Bank.

Erni, C., & Luithi, S. (2001). *Indigenous and tribal peoples in India Desk Review, Project to promote ILO policy on indigenous and tribal peoples*. Geneva: ILO.

Faircloth, S.C., & Tippeconnic, W. (2010). The dropout/graduation crisis among American Indian and Alaska Native students: Failure to respond places the future of native peoples at risk. *The Civil Rights Project/Proyecto Derechos Civiles at UCLA and The Pennsylvania State University Center for the Study of Leadership in American Indian Education.*

Fombonne, E. (2009). Epidemiology of pervasive developmental disorders. *Pediatric Research, 65*(6), 591–598.

Freeman, C., & Fox, M. (2005). *Status and trends in the education of American Indians and Alaska Natives* (NCES 2005-108). Washington, DC: U.S. Department of Education, National Center for Education Statistics.

Frize, M., Kenny, D., & Lennings, C. (2008). The relationship between intellectual disability, indigenous status and risk of reoffending in juvenile offenders on community orders. *Journal of Intellectual Disability Research, 52*(6), 510–519.

Fuchs, E., & Havighurst, R. J. (1972). *To live on this earth: American Indian Education.* Doubleday: Garden City, NY.

Gallagher, B. T. (2000). Teaching (Native) Americans. *The Nation, 270,* 36–38.

Gautam, V. (2003). *Education of tribal children in India and the issues of medium of instruction: A Janshala experience.* Delhi, India: UN/Government Janshala Programme.

Gee, V., & O'Neill, M. T. (2001). *Prenatal statistics in Western Australia, 2001.Nineteenth annual report of the Western Australian midwives' notification system.* Perth, WA: Department of Health.

Glasson, E. J., Sullivan, S. G., Hussain, R., & Bittles, A. H. (2005). An assessment of intellectual disability among Aboriginal Australians. *Journal of Intellectual Disability Research, 49*(8), 626–634.

Gracey, M., Williams, P., & Houston, S. (1997). Environmental health conditions in remote and rural Aboriginal communities in Western Australia. *Australian and New Zealand Journal of Public Health, 21,* 511–8.

Grantham-McGregor, S. (2002). Linear growth retardation and cognition. *Lancet, 359,* 564.

Hall, G., & Patrinos, H. (2010). Indigenous peoples, poverty and development. *Manuscript report.*

Harris, K. R., & Bucens, I. K. (2003). Prevalence of fetal alcohol syndrome in the top end of the Northern Territory. *Journal of Paediatrics and Child Health, 39,* 528–33.

Helme, S., & Lamb, S. (2011). *Closing the school completion gap for indigenous students* (Resource Sheet No. 6). Canberra: Australian Institute of Health and Welfare & Family Studies.

Helps, Y. L., & Harrison, J. E. (2004). *Reported injury mortality of Aboriginal and Torres Strait Islander people in Australia, 1997–2000. Australian Institute of Health and.* Adelaide: Welfare.

Herring, R. D. (1994). Substance use among Native American Indian youth: A selection review of causality. *Journal of Counseling and Development, 72,* 578–584.

Hetzel, B. S. (1983). Iodine deficiency disorders (IDD) and their eradication. *Lancet, ii,* 1126–8.

Health Organization (2002). Prevention of Blindness and Visual Impairment, Causes of blindness and visual impairment. Atlas child and adolescent Mental healt resources globa concerns implications for the future. World Health Organization.

Hirschfeld, A. J., & Fleshman, J. K. (1969). An unusually high incidence of salt-losing congenital adrenal hyperplasia in the Alaskan Eskimo. *Journal of Pediatrics, 75,* 492–49.

House, J. D. (2003). A longitudinal assessment of cognitive-motivational predictors of the grade performance of American Indian/Alaska Native students. *International Journal of Instructional Media, 30,* 303–314.

Huff, D. (1997). *To live heroically: Institutional racism and American Indian education.* Albany: State University of New York Press.

ILO. (2001). *Traditional occupations of indigenous and tribal peoples: Emerging trends.* Geneva: ILO.

International Youth Foundation. (2000). *The situation of children and youth in Oaxaca, Mexico.* Mexico country study. International Youth Federation.

Jeffries, R. B., Hollowell, M., & Powell, T. (2004). Urban American Indian students in a no punitive alternative high school. *American Secondary Education, 32,* 63–78.

Joe, J. R. (1997). American Indian children with disabilities: The impact of culture on health and education services. *Families, Systems & Health, 15*(3), 251–261.

Jones, J., Ritenbaugh, C., Spence, A., Hayward, A. (1991). Severe combined immunodeficiency among the Navajo: characterization of phenotypes, epidemiology and population genetic. *Humen Biology, 63*, 669–682.

Kratli, S. (2001). *Education provision to nomadic pastoralists: A literature review*. Institute of Development Studies (IDS): Environment Team. http://www.eldis.org/pastoralism.

Kumar, A. (2008). *Universal primary education among tribals in Jharkhand*. Ranchi, Jharkhand: Xavier Institute of Social Service.

Larsen, P.B. (2003). Indigenous and tribal children: Assessing child labour and education challenges (Child Labour and Education Working Paper). A Joint IPEC & INDISCO-COOP Publication.

Leonard, H., Petterson, B., De Klerk, N., Zubrick, S. R., Glasson, E., Sanders, R., et al. (2005). Association of socio-demographic characteristics of children with intellectual disability in Western Australia. *Social Science & Medicine, 60*, 1499–513.

Lewis, J. (2001). *The Batwa Pygmies of the Great Lakes Region*. London: Minority Rights Group International.

Loeb, M., & Eide, A. H. (2004). *Living conditions among people with activity limitations in Malawi* (SINTEF Report No. STF78 A044511). Oslo: SINTEF Health Research.

Lopez, M. (2007, May). *Integration of indigenous peoples' perspectives in country development processes* (Review of selected CCAs and UNDAFs, No. 2). Prepared for the Secretariat of the United Nation Permanent Forum on Indigenous Issues.

Lumsden, S. (2008, September 30). Making indigenous poverty history. *Journey*. Queensland Uniting Church.

Lund, S. (2000). Adult education and indigenous peoples in Norway. In L. King (Coordinator). *International survey on adult education for indigenous people*. UNESCO.

Martinez, M. A. (2000). *Review of developments: Indigenous children and youth, item 4* (Working Group on Indigenous Populations, Report: E/CN4/Sub.2/2000/24). Geneva: Office of the United Nations High Commissioner for Human Rights.

Maybury-Lewis, D. (2007). *Indigenous peoples, ethnic groups and the state*. Needham, MA: Allyn & Baker.

Mendola, P., Sherry, G., Gutter, S., & Rice, D. (2002). Environmental factor associated with a spectrum of neurodevelopment deficits. *Mental Retardation and Developmental Disabilities Research Reviews, 8*, 188–197.

Miles, M. (1997). Afghan children and mental retardation: Information, advocacy and prospects. *Disability Rehabilitation, 19*, 496–500.

Moncher, M. S., Holden, G. W., & Trimble, J. E. (1990). Substance abuse among Native-American youth. *Journal of Consulting and Clinical Psychology, 58*, 408–415.

Moran, R., Rampey, B. D., Dion, G., & Donahue, P. (2008). *National Indian education study 2007: Part I: Performance of American Indian and Alaska Native students as Grades 4 and 8 on NAEP 2007 reading and mathematics assessments (NCES 2008–457)*. Washington, DC: National Center for Education Statistic, Institute of Education Sciences, U.S. Department of Education.

Mullick, S. B. (2002). Tribal domestic working women in Delhi, India (pp. 3–4). *IWGIA Newsletter.*

Neisworth, J. T., & Bagnato, S. J. (2005). DEC recommended practices: Assessment. In S. Sandall, M. L. Hemmeter, B. J. Smith, & M. E. McLean (Eds.), *DEC recommended practices: A comprehensive guide for practical application in early intervention/early childhood special education* (pp. 45–69). Longmont, CO: Sopris West.

NSW Department of Juvenile Justice. (2003). *NSW young people in custody health survey—Key findings report*. Sydney: NSW Department of Juvenile Justice. ISBN 0734765185.

NSW Department of Juvenile Justice. *Disability action plan 2004–2006* (p. 5.). Sydney: NSW.

Olatawura, M. O. (2005). Mental health care for children: The needs of African countries. *World Psychiatry, 4*, 159.

Olusanya, B. O. (2010). Is undernutrition a risk factor for sensor neural hearing loss in early infancy? *British Journal of Nutrition, 103*, 1296–1301.

Omigbodun, O. (2004). Psychosocial issues in a child and adolescent psychiatric clinic. *Social Psychiatry and Psychiatric Epidemiology, 39*, 667–672.

Omigbodun, O. (15 th to 18 th December, 2008). WAHO/IDRC Workshop on Improvement of Maternal and Neonatal Health in West Africa. Cotonou, Benin.

Palma-Sealza, L., & Sealza, S. (2000). *Child labor involving indigenous peoples: The case of a Manobo community in Bukidnon province*. Draft document for ILO-INDISCO & IPEC, Manila.

Partridge, W. L., Jorge, E. (1996, June 30–July 2). *Including the excluded: Ethnodevelopment in Latin America*. Paper presented at the Annual World Bank Conference on Development in Latin America and the Carribean, Bogotá, Colombia.

Pastor-Soler, N. M., Rafi, M. A., Hoffman, J. D., Wenger, D. A., et al. (1994). Metachromatic leukodystrophy in the Navajo Indian population: A splice site mutation in Intron 4 of the aryl-sulfatase A gene. *Human Mutation, 4*, 199–207.

Powers, K., Potthoff, S. J., Bearinger, L. H., & Resnick, M. D. (2003). Does cultural programming improve educational outcomes for American Indian youth? *Journal of American Indian Education, 42*, 17–49.

Psacharopoulos, G. (1994). Returns to investment in education: A global update. *World Development, 22*(9), 1325–43.

Reyes-Boquiren, R. (2001). *Child labour among indigenous peoples: The case of the indigenous communities in the Cordillera Region, Philippines*. Draft document for ILO-INDISCO.

Richman, N. (1993). After the flood. *American Journal of Public Health, 83*, 1522–4.

Riede, P. (2001). More than a mascot. *School Administrator, 58*, 27–33.

Salazar, M. C. (1998). Child work and education in Latin America. In M. C. Salazar & W. A. Glasinovich (Eds.), *Child work and education: Five case studies from Latin America*. Florence: UNICEF.

Schinke, S. P., Tepavac, L., & Cole, K. C. (2000). Preventing substance use among Native American youth: Three-year results. *Addictive Behaviors, 25*, 387–397.

Scholl, T. O., & Hediger, M. L. (1994). Anemia and iron-deficiency anemia: Complication of data on pregnancy outcome. *American Journal and Clinical Nutrition, 59*, 492S–500S.

Shaughnessy, L., Doshi, S. R., & Jones, S. E. (2004). Attempted suicide and associated health risk behaviors among Native American high school students. *Journal of School Health, 74*, 177–182.

Sherman, L. (2002). To realize the dream: Research sheds new light on how educators can fulfill the boundless promise that minority children bring to school with them. *Northwest Education Magazine, 8*, 2–9.

Shrout, P., & Newman, S. (1989). Design of two-phase prevalence surveys of rare disorders. *Biometrics, 45*, 549–55.

Singleton, R., Helgerson, S. D., Snyder, R. D., O'Conner, P. J., Nelson, S., Johnson, S. D., et al. (1990). Neuropathy in Navajo children: Clinical and epidemiologic features. *Neurology, 40*, 363–361.

Sommer, A., & West, K. P. (1997). The duration of the effects of vitamin A supplementation. *American Journal of Public Health, 87*, 467–9.

Stiffman, A. R., Alexander-Eitzman, B., Silmere, H., Osborne, V., & Brown, E. (2007). From Early to late adolescence; American Indian youths' behavioral trajectories and their major influences. *Journal of the American Academy of Child and Adolescent Psychiatry, 46*, 849–858.

The Senate Community Affairs References Committee. (2005). *Protecting vulnerable children: A national challenge* (Second report on the inquiry into children in institutional or out-of-home care), US Senate.

Thorburn, M. J., Desai, P., & Durkin, M. (1991). A comparison of the key informant and the community survey methods in the identification of childhood disability in Jamaica. *Epidemiology, 1*, 255–61.

Torzillo, P. J., Hanna, J. N., Morey, F., Gratten, M., Dixon, J., & Erlich, J. (1995). Invasive pneumococcal disease in Central Australia. *Medical Journal of Australia, 162*, 182–6.

U.S. Department of the Interior, National Park Service. *National NAGPRA: Indian reservations in the continental United States map index* [cited 2005 June 22]. Retrieved from: http://www.nps.gov/nagpra/DOCUMENTS/ResMapIndex.htm.

UNESCO. (1999). *Examination of the reports and responses received in the sixth consultation of member states on the implementation of the convention and recommendation against discrimination in education.* Executive Board, 156EX/21.

USAID. (1997). *Education of Indigenous girls in Latin America: Closing the gap.* Information Bulletin, USAID, Office of Women in Development.

Viteri, F. E. (1998). Prevention of iron deficiency. In E. T. Kennedy, A. Horwitz, & Committee on Micronutrient Deficiencies, Institute of Medicine (Eds.), *Prevention of micronutrient deficiencies: Tools for policymakers and public health workers* (pp. 45–102). Washington, DC: National Academic Press.

Vraniak, D. (1997). Mapping contexts for supporting American Indian Families of young with disabilities. *Families, Systems & Health, 15*(3), 283–300.

Whitbeck, L. B., Mansoo, Y., Johnson, K. D., Hoyt, D. R., & Walls, M. L. (2008). Diagnostic prevalence rates from early to mid-adolescence among indigenous adolescents: First results from a longitudinal study. *Journal of the American Academy of Child and Adolescent Psychiatry, 47*, 890–900.

World Health Organization. (1996). *Control of hereditary diseases* (World Health Organization Technical Report Series 865). Geneva: WHO.

Wright, D. G. (1970). The unusual skeletal findings of the Kuskokwim syndrome. *Births Defects, 6*, 16–24.

Yeo, R., & Moore, K. (2003). Including disabled people in poverty reduction work: "Nothing about us without us." In *World Development* (Vol. 31, No. 3. pp. 571–590). Great Britain: Elsevier Science.

Chapter 2
Key Terms

2.1 Culture

Everyone has a culture. Culture and language provide people with ways to organize their thoughts, communicate with others, and manage the world. It is through culture that we think, feel, behave, and manage our reality (Shweder 1991). Culture allows us to know who we are, define what is meaningful, communicate with others, and manage our environment. Just as we use our eyes to see the world, we use our culture to understand our world.

In cross-cultural psychology, culture has been described as a fuzzy set, i.e., a term on which there is lack of agreement regarding its definition, conceptualization, and operationalization. The word "culture" originates from the Latin word *cultura*, which means "to till or cultivate." Talor (1871) defined culture as "that complex whole which includes knowledge, belief, arts, morals, laws, customs and any other capabilities and habits acquired as a member of society" (cited in Kim et al. 2006).

When referring to culture, we mean the totality of ideas, values, knowledge, and way of life of a group of people who share a certain historical, religious, racial, linguistic, ethnic, or social background (Henry et al. 1995).

A number of authors have attempted to define culture succinctly. Slaughter et al. (1990) wrote that culture "is the sum total of mores, traditions, and beliefs of how we function, and encompasses other products of human works and thoughts specific to members of an intergenerational group, community, or population" (p. 363). Rehm (1999) takes a slightly different view, defining culture as "a dynamic and negotiated social construction arising from interaction and resulting in shared understandings among people in contact with one another" (p. 66).

Culture is not a variable, quasi-independent variable, or a mere sum of individual characteristics. Culture is an emergent property of individuals interacting with, managing, and changing their environment. Culture represents the collective utilization of natural and human resources to achieve desired outcomes (Kim et al. 2006), and it is usually associated with the study of the past (e.g., history, philosophy, art, literature, language, and crafts).

I. Manor-Binyamini, *School-Parent Collaborations in Indigenous Communities:*   37
Providing Services for Children with Disabilities, DOI 10.1007/978-1-4614-8984-9_2,
© Springer Science+Business Media New York 2014

It is always easier to detect the influence of culture in people other than ourselves. Culture is something to which we have grown so accustomed that we have ceased to notice its effects; nonetheless, it is not surprising that culture has such a profound influence on our behavior. It is a part of our life from inception: our mother's practices during pregnancy, the way we are cared for as infants, the language and sounds that surround us, and the rules that we are taught as we grow up. Culture is a set of value systems that relate strongly to religious beliefs, kinship patterns, social arrangements, communication networks, and regulatory norms of person familial and social conduct (Anderson and Kirkham 1999).

Individuals interpret situations based on their past experience, and these interpretations can never be culture-free. Thus, for example, the rules for touching differ from culture to culture; as a result, the manner in which one interprets an act of touching is necessarily culturally bound. However, cultural beliefs and behaviors are always being influenced by new information and new experiences. Therefore, culture is not static, but rather fluid and dynamic. It encompasses a complex network of meanings, enmeshed within historical, social, economic, and political processes. Given this understanding of culture as a process, and its far-reaching effects, it is clearly impossible to reach an understanding of culture based on a single experience. Rather, learning about one's own and others' cultures is a lifelong process—a journey with multiple destinations.

Cultural characteristics—There are many characteristics that describe a culture, among them communication, space, time, social organization, environmental controls, and biological variations (St Clair and McKenry 1999).

Although communities are not static or planned, societies do have cultural mores, practices, and characteristics which guide human behavior and provide a socialization framework that shapes interactions. Culture is this framework that guides and bounds life practices. Cultural practices, as well as the individual characteristics of the person or family, are likely to influence the interactions between service providers or interventionists and the parents of the children who are the recipients of the services. The task of the service provider, much like that of a gardener, is to individualize interventions, to address families' concerns and priorities, and tailor the services to families' needs and resources. Being sensitive, knowledgeable, and understanding the parents' cultural practices enhances this process and sets the relationship on a constructive course. Lynch and Hanson (1998) stressed that learning about one's own culture, as well as about another's culture, is a process that continues throughout one's lifetime. Bohannan (1989) stated that "the capacity to learn culture is genetic, but the subject matter is not genetic and must be learned by each person in his or her family and social community" and "only part of culture is conscious" (p. 12).

Culture is often confused with race and ethnicity. Originally, the term "race" was intended to denote biological variation, but it currently represents a set of individuals with similar identity factors that include political and social status. Similarly, the term "ethnicity" represents a group of individuals with shared characteristics, such as language, religion, and/or geographical origin (Rehm 1999), which is set apart by boundaries of affiliation (Mink 1997). Rehm (1999) reminds us that most people belong to more than one defined culture, but usually identify themselves with a sole culture.

People usually identify themselves as belonging to a specific culture, yet they do not necessarily reflect or represent all of the characteristics of that culture.

In learning about one's own or another's culture, one must understand how members of that culture communicate. Thus, it is important to know what is considered adequate personal space in that culture, how time is measured, and what are acceptable frameworks in which people may interact. Do members of that culture tend to stay segregated within their own nuclear families or do they interact within the larger extended family and/or community? Answers to these questions can help service providers identify the proper authority figures and facilitate their communication with them. Culturally bound environmental controls also include traditions and beliefs regarding health and illness, and people's place in relation to the environment, namely, whether people believe they control—or are controlled by—the environment (Giger and Davidhizar 2004).

Culture is an anchor that ties an individual to a social community. We do know certain things about culture. Culture influences behavior (Lynch and Hanson 2004). What we choose to do and how we do, it is usually dictated by cultural appropriateness. The way we greet people, how we express our pleasure or displeasure in various situations, what we eat, and what we wear is often a matter of culturally determined norms. The character and appropriateness of interpersonal relationships is usually influenced by the cultural dictates of the community. Culture shapes one's values (Lynch and Hanson 2004). The values that are most important to us are determined (or at least influenced) by our culture(s). We see this clearly, as we look at various cultural groups around the world. The fact that in the United States Anglo European Americans tend to place a high value on individual freedom whereas people from more traditional cultures may have a collective orientation is an example of culturally shaped values (Davis-McFarland and Dowell 2000). Culture acts as a screen for interpreting other cultures (Lynch and Hanson 2004). We view and evaluate unfamiliar cultures through our own cultural lens. Our ability to value other cultures may be related to our ability to expand our cultural horizons to understand and appreciate other cultures. Cultures have some characteristics in common.

Hundreds of definitions of culture can be found in the anthropology literature. In this chapter, culture is broadly defined as a system of learned and shared standards for perceiving, interpreting, and behaving in interactions with others and with the environment. Two inherent assumptions of this definition are that culture is learned and that it is shared. Human beings learn culture from those with whom they interact, beginning at the moment of birth (and some would say before birth). Parents, as well as any others who cared for us as young children, are the formidable teachers of cultural values, beliefs, and behaviors. Values are ideas about what is normal and abnormal, proper and improper, desirable and undesirable, and right and wrong. Values form the basis for our beliefs and behaviors. Culture should be viewed as a system; that is, culture is made up of discrete but interconnected components. A culture system consists of the following elements:

- Normative codes (ways of behaving) such as food practices, religious practices, and child-rearing practices.
- Communication codes (both verbal and nonverbal).

Table 2.1 Collectivist and individualistic value systems

Cultural orientation	Personal characteristics	Behavioral indicator
Individualism	• Self-expression • Assertiveness • Self-advocacy • Self-realization	• Communicating dissatisfaction with services • Viewing services in a manner different from that of the family unit or community • Focusing on the individual's unique set of talents and potential
Collectivism	Is inseparable from the family and community • Self-interest is sacrificed in favor of family—or larger group—interests Group activities are dominant	An individual may not accept either transportation assistance or employment from outside his or her community • Suggestions for achieving self-sufficiency are not welcomed

Adopted from Sotnik and Jezewski (2005, p. 24)

- Knowledge (information necessary to function as a member of a culture group).
- Problem-solving strategies (how everyday problems are resolved).
- Relationships (family and social).
- Methods of transmitting culture to the young or to new members of the culture group.

Underlying and shaping these elements are the basic values and beliefs of the group. These elements function as a whole. A change in one component, or the introduction of a new or unfamiliar element, can affect other components, as well as the system as a whole (Sotnik and Jezewski 2005, p. 21). A child with disability in the family constitutes a change that affects several of the components presented herein.

Adherence to a collectivist or an individualistic value system also characterizes the manner in which people perceive their world and behave in it. The framework shown in Table 2.1 indicates several examples of diverse cultural values and potential implications for understanding disability and accepting disability-related supports.

It is important to state that most of the indigenous communities in the world live in a bicultural world. For example, many Native Americans and Alaska Natives live in both the traditional (tribal) and the modern world. Within this bicultural world, a person's values, ideas, and beliefs are constantly influenced by the degree of interaction between the two worlds. How these worlds are negotiated at the individual level is not always obvious. Some Native American families may be very traditional in their spiritual values, but very modern in other respects. Thus, they actively participate in all tribal religious activities, but may also have a successful career on Wall Street. The cultural continuum for Native American families ranges from highly traditional to highly acculturated, with significant number of individuals and families found midrange, that is, with a strong footing in both the Native American culture and the white world culture. The degree of acculturation that results from living in a bicultural world greatly influences Native American families' perceptions of—as well as their responses to—disability.

Most people have multiple cultures. There is racial culture as well as ethnic culture, and other cultures related to gender, religion, age, physical size, socioeconomic status, physical ability, and so on. Children with disabilities belong to a subculture as a result of their diagnoses—the "culture of disability" (Eddey and Robey 2005, p. 70). Their parents, as shown, often belong to a racial, ethnic, or cultural minority. Thus, due to genetics, the environment, or both, these children belong to two minority cultures: ethnicity and disability. Some may also belong to a third culture—that of poverty. If we generally agree that human behavior is shaped by the cultural context in which the individual developed, then the experiences or needs of children with disabilities and of their parents cannot be understood apart from the culture in which these families live. Culture fosters values, norms, attitudes, and perceptions about disabilities, as well as the goals parents set for their children, including the framework or agenda for development. Nsamenang (2000) refers to these as the "*cultural curriculum*." In other words, culture also mediates children's and parents' views of the intervention process, the extent to which they are willing to seek education or therapy, and which types of education and therapy they consider valid and desirable. It also defines the nature of disability, provides the diagnostic labels, and formulates social policy and priorities regarding services and support for those with disabilities. Hence, the concept of culture and familiarity with the indigenous community's culture are crucial to the success of the professional intervention. This is particularly true in the context of schools where the strained relationships between professionals and parents of children with disabilities could be mollified or at least diffused by understanding the parents' culture.

It should be understood that culture is only one of many elements that parents use to define themselves and their children; another important key concept is *indigenous knowledge*.

2.2 Indigenous Knowledge

> That which is learned through the mouth is forgotten
> It is through the soul that we learn.
> The soul repeats it in the heart, not in the mind,
> And only then do we know what to do.
> (Manual Arias Sojob: Interview with Guiteras Holmes, 1961)

Most of us in the Western world are accustomed to learning about the world primarily through our senses of sight and hearing. Despite a few interesting experiments in the education of the "lower" senses, the senses of smell, taste, and touch have not been accorded a place in mainstream Western education. These senses tend to be associated with either "savagery" or sensualism. When we look across cultures, however, a different sensory picture emerges, in which each of the senses plays a vital role in the acquisition of knowledge of the world. The following are only a few some of the many examples that exist around the world. For the Desana people of the Colombian rainforest, the sound of every bird call, the color and scent of every flower, the taste of every fruit is imbued with a message about the social and cosmic order. The Desana remind us that knowledge comes from the full-bodied experience and interpretation of our environment (Classen 1999, p. 269). Another example is the significance of water for some of the indigenous communities in the world, such as the Nimiipuu. The Nimiipuu live in the basins of the Snake and Columbia Rivers. The Nimiipuu have maintained an indigenous knowledge system of water (kúus), which has an ideological and material importance in Nimiipuu cosmology and for everyday survival. From an ideological perspective, water is home to powerful spirits, while from a material perspective, water is used for medicine and healing purposes. According to Nimiipuu cosmology, eddies and confluences of free-flowing rivers and waterfalls are thought of as the homes of spirits; thus, the Nimiipuu see dams as killing streams. Similar to their regard for fish, they do not consider all water sources to be the equal in either importance or preference. Springs possess the purest, strongest, and most spiritually powerful water and are used in the ritual sweathouse, where the water is poured on hot rocks. Cold flowing water from high mountain streams is less preferred than spring water, but is considered "better" than water that runs at lower elevations, with less velocity, and at higher temperatures. Nimiipuu water priorities reflect their adaptive capacity, since spring water most often has fewer pollutants than does water at lower velocities and higher temperatures, which makes the latter a better habitat for pathogens. Water (kúus) and salmon (léwliks) are therefore essential to the life of Nimiipuu (Colombi 2012).

There is no curriculum for the knowledge presented in these examples, because for most of these communities it has been communicated via an oral tradition, passed down from generation to generation, from grandparents to grandchildren and from parents to children, in the family, and as part of community life. This knowledge cannot really be separated from life; it is ingrained in all aspects of life.

This is also true regarding all other areas of life in most indigenous communities. For example, the Pygmies of Central Africa have traditionally been closely attached to the rainforest. They were the "Forest People," and the forest was the source of their religion, livelihood, and protection. They used to lead a nomadic life in camps of 30–40 families, which maintained regular links and exchanges with each other. Their mostly egalitarian and horizontal society acknowledged the wisdom of elders who preserved the community's knowledge of the sites, plants, animals, ghosts and spirits, as well as their entire cultural heritage (rituals, music, dances, holy sites) and practices (pharmacopeia, hunting, and fishing).

Another example of a form of indigenous knowledge pertains to traditional healing, which is based on a holistic approach towards both the intervention and the person to be treated (Ong et al. 2005). Traditional healing considers the whole person and acts simultaneously on the physical, mental, spiritual, and emotional levels. Knowledge of traditional medicine methods is the domain of specialists who assume traditional roles. This knowledge has been passed on from father to son for thousands of years throughout history. One manifestation of such traditional knowledge is the role of the *medicine man*, as described in various indigenous societies (Kiev 1964). The medicine man diagnoses illnesses and treats them. He prophesies,

Table 2.2 Unique attributes of indigenous knowledge

Indigenous knowledge
• Natural resource
• Local knowledge—unique to a given culture or society
• Basis for local-level decision making in agriculture, healthcare, food preparation, education, natural resource management, and a host of other activities in rural communities
• Passed down from one generation to the next
• Lacks a canonical foundation in written form
• Unofficial, un-institutionalized system
• Applicable knowledge—relies almost exclusively on intuition combined with sensory evidence
• Closed and isolated system, characterized by a lack of awareness of other possible ways to view the world
• Encompasses cultural traditions, values, beliefs, and worldviews of local peoples
• Holistic and inclusive form of knowledge
• Indigenous knowledge and peoples are disappearing all over the world as a direct result of the pressures of modernization

locates lost belongings, and escorts the spirits of the dead to their destiny in the world beyond. He exposes criminals and punishes them, sways the weather, and, in hunter societies, guarantees bountiful prey. The medicine man embodies the community's mythology, theology, and cosmology and protects them from the forces of evil. From these sources it appears that in premodern societies the medicine man was important in religious and political terms, and was perceived as the preserver of the community's cultural heritage. Given its status of unofficial, un-institutionalized, pluralistic, and heterogeneous system, the trove of traditional knowledge tends to dissipate due to the absence of a written canon by which to convey this knowledge. The unique attributes of indigenous knowledge that were introduced through the examples provided here are summarized in Table 2.2.

In many countries in the world, there is growing recognition of the importance of indigenous knowledge, some of which is in danger, as expressed in the term Bio-piracy. *Bio-piracy* is the act of appropriating indigenous peoples' knowledge of nature and exploiting it or commercial gain without obtaining permission from or providing compensation to the indigenous people themselves. Critics of this use of indigenous knowledge, such as Greenpeace, claim these practices contribute to inequality between developing countries rich in biodiversity and the developed countries that act as hosts to biopirating companies. Earth-based resources used by indigenous and traditional peoples include medicinal uses of plants, fish, animals, and other resources located on lands, rivers, and seas. This knowledge stems from indigenous peoples' long-lasting attachment to their environment and a history of maintaining that environment over millennia in various places around the world. There are a number of key examples of bio-piracy in the literature. The case against W.R. Grace's patent on the neem tree is one of the most cited examples. Yet, this case is unique in that there exist written Sanskrit sources supporting the indigenous community's claim to earlier knowledge of the neem's medicinal attributes. However, most indigenous communities rely on oral—rather than—written histories. This is the case for example in Australia. As one of the megadiverse regions of the world, Australia is home to numerous flora and fauna, which are being explored by corporate scientists. Thus, the Western Australia smokebush, which has long been used by Aboriginal people for medicinal purposes, is now being examined for its active ingredient, concurvane, which could prove effective in combating HIV (Christie 2001).

The disappearance of indigenous knowledge is also closely tied to the lack of protection of indigenous peoples' rights. Coupled with an ever-increasing external demand for natural resources found on indigenous territories and projects that have a detrimental effect on the environments and natural resources of indigenous communities, the absence of protective rights leads to increased poverty and social exclusion. Climate change is also a crucial issue that may well affect indigenous peoples' chances of survival. Indigenous communities have lived in harmony with nature for centuries. Unfortunately, in many countries, traditional indigenous knowledge of the environment and of medicine is in danger of being lost, just when such knowledge is desperately needed in order to restore balance to the environment after centuries of abuse at human hands. However, at the same time that indigenous knowledge is disappearing in some countries, there is a growing trend around the world of recognizing indigenous knowledge and its importance.

Evidence of the allure which indigenous knowledge holds for theorists and practitioners alike lies in multiple arenas. New international and national institutions sponsor inquiries into indigenous knowledge. Funding agencies attempt to incorporate issues related to indigenous knowledge in their financial activities (CIDA, IDRC, UNESCO, and the World Bank, as examples). Newsletters, journals, and other modes of communication that act as a mouthpiece for such organizations emphasize the significance of indigenous knowledge. In numerous conferences, scholars and development professionals discuss the merits of indigenous knowledge and deploy a new populist rhetoric to assert the relevance of indigenous knowledge in development planning. The words of Warren et al. (1993, p. 2) highlight the recent shift:

> Ten years ago, most of the academics working in the area of indigenous knowledge represented anthropology, development sociology, and geography. Today… important contributions are also being made in the fields of ecology, soil science, veterinary medicine, forestry, human health, aquatic science, management, botany, zoology, agronomy, agricultural economics, rural sociology, mathematics,… fisheries, range management, information science, wildlife management, and water resource management.

Therefore, many researchers, professionals, and specialists working in indigenous communities agree that development planning strategies must incorporate indigenous knowledge. The integration of this knowledge in this context would enable a more culturally sensitive and a relationship-oriented model in the area of care, for example, thus facilitating the establishment of institutional level support services for indigenous communities. Such a framework would be more appropriate than existing ones and would be able to integrate preventative interventions and health promotion.

One of the many examples presented by Kleinman (1980), a pioneer of research of traditional medicine in multicultural societies, is especially interesting, as it sheds light on the complexity of indigenous knowledge. Following a field study he conducted in Taiwan, he pointed out that there were three treatment systems operating concurrently. The three systems he identified—professional, folk, and traditional—were based on differing principles of diagnosis, classification, and treatment. "The professional system" relied on the principles of science. Authorized doctors would primarily utilize biochemical means to treat patients, with the aid of supporting specialists. This was the most dominant and institutionalized system, which received financial support and professional recognition from the government. The "folk system," on the other hand, was an amateur, unofficial system. Individuals either provided themselves with initial treatment or were cared for by their families or acquaintances. This was the most common system: it served for defining the individual's problem, it provided the lion's share of the treatment, and it constituted the focal point of the individual's decision making and engagement. The folk system dealt not only with the healing of sickness but also with its prevention. It was tied in with the other two systems—the professional and the traditional—which were themselves sometimes disengaged from each other. Despite its importance, it received little research attention, especially compared to the traditional system, which was considered dramatic and exotic. According to Kleinman, the traditional system was a specialist system even though it lacked bureaucratic specialists and a written canonical basis. It functioned as an unofficial, un-institutionalized, naturalistic, and heterogeneous system. Its agents and their actions were often associated with a sacred sector that operated in relation to supernatural spirits, and a secular sector that operated at the physical level and concentrated on areas such as herbal medicine and massage. In most cases the sacred sector received more research attention than did the secular one. The traditional healer was portrayed as relying on supernatural elements—spirits, ghosts, ancestors, and other supernatural entities, and as being part of an existing religious tradition.

It is important to note that at this point in time we are at a crucial crossroads regarding the preservation of indigenous knowledge, since most indigenous communities have already been affected by deep processes of transformation, such as urbanization, culturalization, and modernization, processes which inevitably affect indigenous knowledge. These communities are at a junction, between tradition and modernity, between change and preservation; consequently, any measures taken in order to get to know, preserve, and publish indigenous knowledge are of great value. For instance, indigenous Knowledge and Development Monitor is a publication of and for the international community of people who are interested in indigenous knowledge. It is produced by three major international centers on indigenous knowledge: CIRAN—the Centre for International Research and Advisory Networks in the Netherlands; CIKARD—the Center for Indigenous Knowledge for Agricultural and Rural Development in Iowa, United States; and LEAD—the Leiden Ethnosystems and Development Program in the Netherlands. These international centers assist and follow the activities of regional and national centers in Nigeria (ARCIK), Philippines (REPPIKA), Brazil, Burkina Faso, Ghana, Kenya, Indonesia, Mexico, South Africa, Uruguay, and Venezuela.

Indigenous knowledge is not the only aspect of indigenous communities that is in danger of disappearing. Keep in mind that globally, there is a great deal of diversity among indigenous communities and, correspondingly, their knowledge troves are also diverse. Each indigenous community and each individual within a community must be approached as unique. At the same time, themes emerge from shared experiences of genocide, bondage, colonization, and alienation, difficulties which have affected and continue to affect indigenous peoples worldwide. I chose to focus on one central subject out of many, namely, lands and territories.

2.3   Lands and Territories

The issue of lands and territories is a primary axis from which a long line of issues derives, some of which create longstanding conflicts between indigenous communities and the countries in which they live. This type of conflict extends to nearly all parts of the world.

Indigenous peoples have a special twofold attachment to their ancestral lands and territories. Spiritually, land plays a fundamental role in indigenous and tribal cultural identities, cosmologies, and beliefs, while on a practical and material level, it is their most essential resource, on which they depend for their livelihood.

For most indigenous peoples the attitude towards land is not limited to its value as property. It is the land that binds the community to all areas of life; therefore, the meanings attributed to it are deeper. Theirs is a holistic and communal conception of land, one which nourishes and sustains the group's identity. The contours of the tribal panorama define the identity and affiliation of the indigenous peoples and bind them to the land. This is a sustainable, honorable, mutual, balancing relationship: land is home, culture, spirituality, tradition, ancestral burial grounds, and environment.

At the same time, indigenous peoples are deeply dependent on land resources, through highly adaptive livelihood systems and practices. Their connection to the land was ratified at ILO Convention 1969, which recognized the right of ownership and possession of indigenous and tribal peoples over the lands they have traditionally occupied. Although some progress was made since then, the issue of land rights remains a highly contested topic. Even in countries with progressive legislation, indigenous communities face considerable challenges in terms of protecting their traditional territories. Recognition of indigenous and tribal land rights remains a complicated field in terms of its technical, economic, and political dimensions. Control of place creates a right to material and cultural resources, and to its instrumental, moral, and aesthetic knowledge (Castree 2004).

Dispossession of land and natural resources is a major human rights problem for indigenous peoples. They have in so many cases been pushed out of their traditional areas to give way to the economic interests of other more dominant groups and large-scale development initiatives, acts which tend to destroy their lives and cultures rather than improve their situation. Large-scale extraction of natural resources such as logging, mining, dam construction, oil drilling, and pipeline construction have had very negative impacts on the livelihoods of indigenous pastoralist and hunter-gatherer communities in Africa. South Africa provides an encouraging example of an attempt to safeguard the land rights of indigenous communities.

The struggle for land is part of a larger effort of indigenous peoples all over the world to secure human rights.

A proper examination of the issue of land struggles and recognition of rights requires a comparative approach, studying countries individually first and then comparing the findings, to create a common language that can serve as an instrument for diagnosing common issues. In other words, such a comparison would set the stage for significant research to be conducted within each country, in order to allow the findings to highlight the main issues and thus provide an overall perspective. From this vantage point, larger structures could be identified and outlined, forming a basis from which to draw more general lessons (Hague and Harrop 2001).

Here I present one example of such study, which compares the types and levels of recognition granted to indigenous communities around the world, ranging from total lack of recognition in a colonial regime to transformative recognition. The various levels of recognition are catalogued according to types of governments and the types of policies and the quality of state-indigenous relations that correspond to these levels are also indicated in Table 2.3. Based on these measures, it is possible to rate each country's attitude towards its indigenous peoples. However, it is important to emphasize that there is a constant dynamic of change, which in many cases creates a disparity between the definitions and the actual state of affairs.

The following comparative summary is based on the levels of recognition presented in the previous table, while emphasizing the insights gleaned from it (Table 2.4).

The comparison between the three countries, Brazil, Australia, and Canada, gives rise to several general insights, some or all of which are important for other indigenous peoples, including:

- There is an apparent difficulty in getting out of the colonial paradigm, after its lengthy and continued existence and as the generator of the state in its current form.
- In all three countries, one cannot point to a policy that coalesces into one type of recognition, but one can identify a main type of recognition. Policies reflect a wide range of types of recognition, and in most cases land policy reflects essential contradictions as it is at times colonial and at times democratic.
- Government support is needed for the various programs to improve the situation of indigenous peoples.
- It is apparent that as time progresses, the programs are getting closer to the indigenous peoples and less assimilative and patronizing.
- Generally, the condition of the indigenous peoples in all countries is worse compared to the other groups in the population. There is still a long way to go— conceptually and consciously, ideationally, governmentally, and financially—until appropriate gains are made, and the past losses, destruction, and oppression are amended.

The example presented demonstrates the engagement with indigenous peoples and their relations with the state they live in. These studies have resulted in a rich and varied body of research (Ivison et al. 2000; Nietzen 2003; Scheinin 2004; Tsosie 2001).

Nevertheless, the actual implementation of even the most far-reaching measures regarding land rights has not significantly improved the socioeconomic conditions

Table 2.3 Diagnostics of the types of recognition, types of policy, and state-indigenous relations

Regime	Types of recognition	Types of policy	State-indigenous relations
Colonialism	No recognition	– Expansion – Takeover – Exploitation – Oppression – Racism	– Killing – Deportation – Dispossession of place and livelihood – Destruction of family – Assimilation
	"Protective" recognition	– Segregation – Oversight, patronage, and limitation of rights	– Citizenship and limited rights
Ethnocracy	Hostile recognition—awareness of the group's existence as a "disturbance" and "threat"	– Spatial inequality in allocation of resources creates ethnic-class stratification – Partial civil rights – Spatial encroachment – Economic, social, cultural discrimination – Declaration of recognition without implementation – Utilization of informal recognition practices – De jure or de facto mechanism of discrimination and inequality, "transience," no right to local vote	– Overt conflict due to antagonism and polarization, may be accompanied by violence – Gray areas and informal development
	Indifferent recognition	– Creeping recognition – Rhetorical recognition – Passive recognition—does not recognize the unique needs of the diagnosed group	– Moderate conflict due to the lack of clear categories – Control, discrimination, marginality
Liberal-democracy	Affirmative recognition	– Integration of traditional law in the legal system – Distributive justice – Planning and development + financing and support – Establishment of indigenous elected body	– Protests and struggles using institutional channels – Achievements accomplished through grassroots struggles

Multicultural democracy	– Political representation on a liberal basis	
	– Constitutional reform/amendment	
	– Apology and reconciliation	
	– Supreme court decisions that promote recognition and rights	
	– Development of a legal construct that addresses needs	
	– Recognition of the group and its needs: danger of marginality	– קצה הדרך רצוי
	– Integration of traditional law in the legal system	
	– Distributive justice	
	– Planning and development+financing and support	
	– Establishment of indigenous tribunal	
	– Transitional justice	– Moderation of the conflict
Transformative recognition	– Political representation on a communal basis	
	– Right to land according to traditional ownership	
	– Right to equal/affirmative and collaborative development	
	– Recognition of difference: accounts for unique economic, social, cultural rights	
	– Prevention of dependence and development of autonomy	
	– Sustainable framework for negotiations over land rights	
	• Development of abilities that accounts for different needs and diversity of each group according to local agendas	
	• Satisfying partnership—move to relations column?	
	• Redistribution of resources, restitution, restoration	
	• Liberty, security, and stability	
	– Formulation of agreement/contract	
	– Provision of the right to self-determination	
	• Mutual fertilization: social–cultural–legal–economic–environmental—move to relations column?	– End of conflict

Adopted from Tzfadia and Roded (2010, p. 10)

Table 2.4 Comparison of Australia, Canada, and Brazil

Country/criterion	Brazil	Australia	Canada
Colonial background	Spanish occupation in the fifteenth century; 500 years of domination and annihilation	British occupation and settlement from the end of the eighteenth century. Ninety percent of aboriginals wiped out	Conquests and settlement beginning from the seventeenth century. Independence from the British in 1867
Civil status	Protégés until 1988	Civil status only from 1948. Referendum in 1967 on constitutional amendment granting civil rights. 1975—law forbidding discrimination and subordination to federal government	Murder, Dispossession of livelihood and land. 1876 Native American Act annulled in 1985. Right to vote granted in 1960
Political representation	One representative elected in 1983	One representative in parliament, representation in states	Most representation is in the indigenous organization. Underrepresentation in parliament
Social and economic situation of indigenous peoples	Indigenous rights are violated, forests cleared, hostile army, invasion, plagues, murder, illegalities. Life expectancy dropped from 48 to 42 in a decade, rash of suicides, 60–80 % have chronic disease, child mortality 13 %	Represent the weak in society by a wide margin: poverty, unemployment, crime, alcoholism, disease, family violence	Indigenous population is younger, less educated, less employed and earn about $8,000 less than nonindigenous. Many do not participate in the work force, crime is rampant
Legal system	Civil law is German. 1988 constitution C 231–2, 67. No proper backing in law. Indigenous matters are directly subordinate to the federation	Customary+verbal testimony and indigenous rights to the land. Constitution promoting indigenous status. Indigenous matters are directly subordinate to the federation	Customary+indigenous Constitution. Backing in law is lacking. Indigenous matters are directly subordinate to the federation

Land policy	1988 constitution—12 % of land recognized as indigenous land, since then process of delineation	Crown lands—terra nullius	1. Legal protection since 1982 and recognition of first rights of indigenous. Ratified in the Constitution Act 35 (1)
	Order 1755—encroaches upon indigenous lands	Mabo ruling in 1992	2. Agreements between tribal leaders and the government
	Only 87 % of indigenous land ratified in 1993	Indigenous land rights law in 1993 Indigenous land tribunal established WICK—1996 1998, 2001—amendments to NTA ILUA	3. In 1998, agreement signed for retreat from 750 mile^2
	Invasion processes, forest clearing, dispossession, and neoliberals with the support of the state	Since 1993, only some claims of ownership have been accepted	
Data about withheld land	10/93 87 % of land sealed. 11.13 % of land given to half the population	Fifteen percent of the land defined as indigenous rights to the land—2.1 % of the population	Indigenous make up 5.24 % of the population and 13 % of the land is registered in their name
Self-government	None	Almost no autonomy. From a representative political body in government to regional decentralization	Autonomous existence. 1999 Inuit 1997 Delgamuukw vs. British Columbia and more
Conflict level	High	Moderate-low	Low
Primary recognition	Hostile-confirming	Affirmative	Transformative

Adopted from Tzfadia and Roded (2010, p. 65)

of indigenous communities relative to the societies they live in and there is still a long way to go to reach full recognition of them and their rights in terms of achieving justice, addressing grievances, and reconciliation.

Despite all the above and alongside the picture presented, it is important to mention that in the past decade there is a trend towards dealing with and discussing restoration of indigenous rights, primarily regarding land and territories, asking forgiveness, compensation, and distributive and transitional justice to the extent of self-government, all under the international aegis of human rights treaties and laws. The change processes are different in each country, but one can see progress towards recognition of injustices caused by settlers and states around the world to indigenous peoples and communities, measures taken towards restorative and transitional justice out of a desire to achieve reconciliation and peace. For example, the federal government announced on Tuesday that it intends to pay $3.4 billion to settle claims that it has mismanaged the revenue in American Native American trust funds, potentially ending one of the largest and most complicated class-action lawsuits ever brought against the United States (New York Times, 8.12.2009).

In September 2007, the Canadian government began to make compensation payments to former students of Native American Residential Schools. By July 2008, the government had received 94,085 applications for the common Experience Payment and issued payments to 66,232 survivors (IntLawGrrls, 11.6.2009).

The New Zealand government has agreed it will pay millions of dollars to a group of indigenous Maori tribes who say they were victims of illegal land seizures and breaches of the Treaty of Waitangi (February 11, 2009 http://Sydney.indymedia.org.au).

2.4   Indigenous Psychology

Two kinds of coexisting contemporary scientific psychologies, namely, indigenous psychology (IP) and Westernized psychology (WP), can be meaningfully distinguished and defined (Yang 2000). These psychologies represent not only two disciplines but also two methodologies which, in turn, produce two distinctive kinds of psychological knowledge. Here I will briefly discuss them and their backgrounds.

The call for the indigenization and development of a psychology that will be socially and culturally valid is a worldwide phenomenon: Africa (Durojaiye 1993; Cameroon, Nsamenang 1995), Americas (Canada, Berry 1974; Latin America, Ardila 1982; Mexico, Diaz-Guerrero 1977), Asia (Hong Kong, Ho 1982; India, Sinha 1984; Japan, Azuma 1984; the Philippines, Enriquez 1993; Taiwan, Yang 2000), Europe (France, Moscovici 1972; Germany, Graumann 1972; Scandinavia, Smedslund 1984), the Middle East (Iran, Moghaddam 1987; Turkey, Kagitcibasi 1984). Many scholars have pointed out that existing psychological theories reflect the values, goals, and issues of the Western world but that they are not generalizable to other societies (Kim and Berry 1993). Azuma (1984) noted that "the development of a truly universal discipline is limited due through Western glasses, he may fail to notice important aspects of the non-Western culture since the schemata for recognizing them are not provided by his science" (p. 49). These scholars point out that each culture should be understood from its own frame of reference, including, its own ecological, historical, philosophical, and religious context.

In human history, there have been three different kinds of psychology: folk psychology (including common-sense psychology), philosophical psychology, and scientific psychology. Folk psychology refers to the ordinary psychological views, assumptions, beliefs, concepts, conjectures, theories, preferences, norms, and practices that have been naturally and gradually acquired through socialization and that are commonly held by the general population of a society (Sinha 2003). In terms of its content and structure, folk psychology does not constitute scientific knowledge, but it can be used as original data for scientific analysis by anthropologists (Dickason 1984) or psychologists (Heider 1958). The folk psychology of a society may be regarded as part of that society's *little tradition*, in Redfield's (1956) sense.

In contrast, philosophical psychology refers to the formal systems of psychological thought, as proposed by a society's philosophers. For example, philosophical psychological theories and concepts are plentiful in Indian philosophy (Sinha 2003), Chinese philosophy (Moore 1967), and Western philosophy (Burnet 1980). Philosophical psychology may be regarded as part of an ethnic or cultural group's *great tradition*, in Redfield's (1956) sense.

Different from both folk and philosophical psychologies, scientific psychology denotes a psychological knowledge system constructed by academic or expert psychologists using a scientific methodology. Nearly all societies have their own naturally developed folk and philosophical psychologies, but only some Western societies have an endogenous scientific psychology. The emergence of these scientific psychologies is a rather late historical phenomenon. They originated in European countries in the late nineteenth century and have flourished since World War II, especially in the United States. European and American scientific psychologies have been continuously imported by non-Western countries (Church and Katigbak 2002).

The first academic movement to advocate the establishment of an indigenous psychology was in the Philippines, in the 1970s, under the leadership of the late Virgilio Enriquez and his followers (Enriquez 1993; Pe-Pua 2006). Since then, other centers of indigenization have appeared, notably in Taiwan, Japan, Korea, India, Cameroon, Hong Kong, Iran, Latin America, Mexico, and New Guinea (Ho et al. 2001, p. 927).

In considering Westernized and indigenous psychology, the latter is the most pertinent approach for the purpose of studying the issue of collaboration between professionals and parents of school children in indigenous communities. Indigenous psychology is an impressive new approach to the study of psychology. By calling attention to the boundaries of mainstream psychology, it reveals other ways of studying human beings. This new approach contradicts the notion of cultural globalization and the dominance of Western culture, and instead offers a system for acquiring psychological knowledge, not in the sense of describing all psychological phenomena in all cultures, but rather in the sense of *strangification*. Thus, by intentionally using the indigenous cultural context as a starting point for its own development, indigenous psychology has created a breakthrough, introducing a new way to increase our understanding of mankind. The premise to which indigenous psychology subscribes, namely, that it, as well as all other approaches to psychology, is rooted in and relative to its particular cultural background, poses a significant challenge to the Western world's traditional self-image of being neutral and objective. With the advent of indigenous psychology, Western psychology has been forced to recognize that it too is a culturally dependent, locally originated indigenous psychology.

In everyday life, people have phenomenological, episodic, and procedural knowledge that enables them to manage their environment, but they may not have the analytical skills to describe how it is achieved. Indigenous psychology advocates examining the knowledge, skills, and beliefs people have about themselves, and studying these aspects in their natural contexts. *It represents a descriptive approach, in which the goal of psychology is to first understand how people function in their natural contexts.* It advocates a transactional model of human functioning that recognizes the importance of agency, meaning, intention, and goals. It recognizes that human psychology is complex, dynamic, and generative. The goal is to create a science that is firmly grounded in the descriptive understanding of human beings.

2.4.1   *Indigenous Psychology—Definitions*

As pointed out by Kim and Berry (1993), indigenous psychology is "the scientific study of human behavior that is native, that is not transported from other regions, and that is designed for its people" (p. 2). After reviewing Kim and Berry's (1993) and several other indigenously oriented psychologists' definitions (Ho 1998), Yang (2000) defined indigenous psychology as "an evolving system of psychological knowledge based on scientific research that is sufficiently compatible with the studied phenomena and their ecological, economic, social, cultural, and historical contexts" (p. 245). He pointed out that all of these definitions "express the same basic goal of developing a scientific knowledge system that effectively reflects, describes, explains, or understands the psychological and behavioral activities in their native contexts in terms of culturally relevant frames of reference and culturally derived categories and theories" (pp. 245–246). Nine characteristics of indigenous psychology can be identified.

First, indigenous psychology emphasizes examining psychological phenomena in a variety of contexts: familial, social, political, philosophical, historical, religious, cultural, and ecological contexts (see additional details in Kim et al. 2006, p. 6).

Second, contrary to popular misconception, indigenous psychology is not simply the study of native peoples, ethnic groups, or people living in Third World countries. Rather, indigenous psychology is an approach that is appropriate for studying any cultural, native, or ethnic group, whether in an economically developing country, a newly industrialized country, or economically developed countries.

Third, indigenous psychology advocates the use of multiple and varied methodologies: philosophical analysis as well as qualitative, quantitative, experimental, and comparative methods.

Fourth, it has been assumed that only natives or insiders of a culture could understand its indigenous and cultural phenomena whereas an outsider could gain only a limited understanding of these. Although a person born and raised in a particular community may have insights into its indigenous phenomena, this is not always the case. Also, an outsider, with an external point of view, can call attention to a phenomenon, which—although treated as natural by a given community—is actually of a cultural nature. An outsider can point out peculiarities, inconsistencies, and blind spots which insiders may have overlooked (Kleinman 1980). According to the framework of indigenous psychology, both internal and external points of view are necessary in order to provide a comprehensive and integrated understanding of psychological phenomena (Kim et al. 2006).

Fifth, people have a complex and sophisticated understanding of themselves and their social world. However, this understanding is often practically- and episodically based, and therefore it might not be sufficiently comprehensive to include an analytical description of the underlying structure or process of understanding the self. Thus, based on episodic and analytic knowledge, general psychology presents psychologists' analytic conceptions, interpretations, and explanations, rather than an accurate representation of human psychology.

Sixth, indigenous psychology is part of a scientific tradition that advocates multiple *perspectives*, but not multiple *psychologies*. Indigenous psychology is part of a scientific tradition which searches for of psychological knowledge rooted in a cultural context. This knowledge can then become the basis of the discovery of psychological universals and can contribute to the advancement of psychology and science.

Seventh, indigenous psychology is identified as a part of the tradition of cultural sciences. In contrast to the assumption underlying physical and biological sciences, according to indigenous psychology, people do not merely react or adapt to the environment, but they are also able to understand and change their environment, other people, and themselves (Bandura 1997).

Eighth, indigenous psychology advocates a linkage between the humanities (philosophy, history, religion, and literature, which focus on human experience) and the social sciences (which focus on analytical knowledge, empirical analysis, and verification).

Ninth, Enriquez (1993) identified two points of departure for conducting research in indigenous psychology: *indigenization from without* and *indigenization from within*. Indigenization from without involves taking existing psychological theories, concepts, and methods and modifying them to fit the local cultural context. In this approach, rather than assuming that a particular theory is universal a priori, researchers modify and adapt psychological theories to integrate them with the local cultural knowledge. Aspects that can be verified across cultures are retained as possible cultural universals. Existing theories in cognitive, developmental, social, and organizational psychology have been modified and extended by indigenous research.

Table 2.5 General psychology and indigenous psychology

General psychology	Indigenous psychology
Seeks to discover decontextualized, mechanical, and universal principles and it assumes that current psychological theories are universal	Questions the universality of existing psychological theories and attempts to discover psychological universals in social, cultural, and ecological contexts
	Represents an approach in which the content (meaning, values, and beliefs) and context (family, society, culture, and ecology) are explicitly incorporated into the research design
Has attempted to develop objective, decontextualized, and universal theories of human behavior, by excluding the subjective aspects of human functioning (consciousness, agency, meaning, and goals)	Advocates examining knowledge, skills, and beliefs people have about themselves and assessing how they function in their familial, social, cultural, and ecological contexts. It emphasizes obtaining a descriptive understanding of human functioning in a cultural context

Indigenization from within means that theories, concepts, and methods are developed internally, and indigenous information is considered to be a primary source of knowledge (Enriquez 1993).

Although both indigenous and general psychology seek to discover universal facts, principles, and laws of human behavior, the starting point of research is different. The following (Table 2.5) summarizes the essential differences between the two types of psychology.

As indicated in Table 2.5, the main goal of developing indigenous psychology is to construct various systems of knowledge based on folk wisdom, in order to help people solve their daily problems more efficiently (Hwang 2010). Hence, this kind of psychology is extremely important to the understanding and collaboration between parents and professionals in the indigenous community. Indigenous psychologists in the world are seeking an alternative to the existing psychological theories and concepts. It has been found that the assumptions that are supposed to be objective, value-free, and universal are in fact enmeshed in Western values—not true universals. Thus, for example, the psychodynamic interpretation of dreams and unconscious drives based on an individual-ego model as well as left-over Freudian interpretations of symbols tied to sex and aggression do little to help in tribal communities with group-oriented egos and a symbology all their own. Jungian archetypes, in contrast, have been helpful in tapping into possible universal constructs that may include spiritual development of indigenes people. Another example is the concept of *guilt*, which has a very different connotation and function in East Asia from its meaning in Western societies (Azuma 1988). In Western psychoanalytic and psychological theories, guilt is presumed to be based on irrational belief, unrealistic fear, or forbidden wishes. Extensive use of guilt is believed to cause later developmental problems in adolescence. In contrast, in East Asia, it is considered appropriate that children feel guilty or indebted towards their parents, for all the devotion, indulgence, sacrifice, and love that they receive from them (Ho 1982). Children feel indebted since they cannot return the love and care that they received from parents. Guilt in East Asia is viewed as an important interpersonal emotion that promotes filial piety, achievement, motivation, and interpersonal closeness.

The extent to which indigenous psychology is different and unique can be seen from the existence of unique phenomena in indigenous communities. Examples of notably unique phenomena are Philipino pakikisama (getting along with or making concessions to others) (Lynch 1973), Japanese amae (presuming and depending upon another's benevolence) (Dai 1956), Chinese face (Ho 1976) and yuan (predestined relational affinity) (Yang and Ho 1988), and Korean woori (an inclusive group: we or us) and cheong (human affection) (Choi and Kim 2003). Given that these and other culturally unique psychological phenomena have never been studied in Western psychology, there are no relevant Western theories, concepts, methods, and tools available for non-Western psychologists to adopt in investigating them. This means that these local populations have to rely upon themselves to conceptualize and theorize about these local phenomena and design proper methods and tools for assessing them. This is a perfect way to wean local psychologists from their overdependence on Western psychology. They themselves have to develop innovative indigenized theories, concepts, and methods for the systematic study of each of the unique phenomena in their respective societies.

Every indigenous population has different primary psychological manifestations that need to be understood by those who come in contact with them. Thus, for example, while there are many specific clinical health issues that have to be understood in working with the indigenous populations of North America, the two most prominent problems are the high rates of alcoholism and suicide. To demonstrate the importance of recognizing unique contextual phenomena, I will elaborate upon the example of suicide among Native Americans.

It is generally accepted concept that the population of Native Americans as a group shows suicide rates higher than those of the general population, although the estimated rates vary from double the rate to a slightly higher rate compared to the national US average (McIntosh and Santos 1981; Webb and Williard 1975). The literature on Native American suicide indicates that the trend on this population is similar to that of the general population, in that the number of suicide attempts is higher among women, while the number of successful attempts is higher among the men. In the years 2002–2006, the highest US suicide rates were among Native Americans with 16.25 suicides per 100,000 (Hader et al. 2012).

Over the last 45 years, many tribal-specific patterns of suicide have been documented, e.g., the Navajo demonstrate a very low rate of suicide (Miller and Schoenfeld 1971; Miller 1979), whereas the Shoshone-Bannock demonstrate a very high rate (Dizmang 1968). Factors associated with Southwestern Native Americans adolescent suicidal ideation have been researched by Novins et al. (1999), and important findings in this study revealed that suicidal ideation was linked to a friend's suicidal behavior, feeling unsupported by family and friends, and a depressive symptomatology. In the study of the Pueblo people, the tribe was characterized as maintaining strong family and community ties, and suicidal ideation was associated with not having both biological parents in the home and with an increase in stressful life events over the last 6 months.

Unique psychological manifestations also require a unique response for the population. Such responses are described and recorded, for example, in their article *Suicide Prevention: A Culture-Specific Model* (LaFromboise and Lewis 2008).

One particular study that should be brought to the attention of researchers of indigenous psychology describes the Zuni youth suicide prevention program, which was developed as an excellent culture-specific model and focused on the development of Zuni life skills (LaFromboise and Lewis 2008). Through collaboration of tribal elders and an external (native) psychological researcher, a model was set in place. It involved the development of specific skill building exercises practiced in a classroom setting by school age children. A 3-year follow-up of tribal suicide statistics demonstrated its effectiveness, as the number of suicides dropped to zero. The model's structure is outlined here.

1. Develop a needs assessment tool within the cultural group, devised by tribal elders and the community, with the assistance of the research team.
2. Present the findings back to the tribal elders, and further discuss their significance.
3. Select the most appropriate culture-specific protocol for implementing the plan.
4. Create an educational component/curricula.
5. Train the tribal staff and teachers to use the curricula, and identify high-risk individuals.
6. Implement the educational model, with follow-up referrals to other mental health staff, while providing feedback to the planning committee.
7. Conduct follow-ups at different time intervals (longitudinal) to interpret the ongoing data and final data, and implement any changes needed. In the particular case of the Zuni youth program, yearly check-ins were held with appropriate advocacy to ensure continuity with staff, faculty, school administration, and tribal leader turn-over.

This model represents an initial step, in terms of pertinent solution-oriented research, since the issue of mental health among Native Americans has not been sufficiently studied. Their Worldviews regarding mental illness and healing have been frequently ignored in the psychological and psychiatric literature. It was only in the early 1990s, for instance, that the American Psychiatric Association began placing a greater emphasis on investigating this ethnic group's understanding of mental illness, and systematically incorporating relevant information in its publications (Mezzich et al. 1996).

Although current psychological practices strive to advocate and promote the wellbeing of indigenous people, the methods utilized by psychologists have historically failed to take into account the beliefs about health and healing held by this population. Native Americans and Alaska Natives, as many other indigenous peoples throughout the world, understand "wellness" holistically, that is, as a combination of physical, mental, emotional, and spiritual elements (Patel 1995; Rice 2003). Illness is perceived as a sign of imbalance among these basic elements, brought about by ancestral spirits, bad spirits, and witchcraft. Healing practices, on the other hand, attempt to restore the natural balance of soul, mind, and body, through spiritual ceremonies and herbal remedies prescribed by community elders and cultural healers (Poonwassi and Charter 2005). Treatment for mental illness also revolves around storytelling, teaching and sharing circles, sweat lodges, and vision quests (Poonwassi and Charter 2005).

Finally, the question occupying many researchers in the field of psychology today is: "Is indigenous psychology a discipline?"

In Webster's II New Riverside University Dictionary, discipline is defined as "a branch of knowledge" (p. 383). According to this definition, indigenous psychology may be considered a distinct discipline from psychological science, because it generates different kinds of psychological knowledge. Shams (2002) portrayed indigenous psychology as an independent discipline. (Yang 2012, p. 12–16) presents the following six characteristics of IP as proof that it is an independent discipline.

1. IP uses Cultural Basis of Knowledge: It is in this sense that IP knowledge has its own native cultural roots or sources. It is a kind of culturally embedded knowledge.
2. This mono cultural knowledge tends to be emic in the sense that it is culture-specific, rather than culture-general (or universal).
3. The IP knowledge system has the Euro-American native culture as its indigenous root and is produced through Western theories, concepts, methods, and tools as if it were universally or cross-culturally applicable.
4. The IP knowledge system is highly indigenously contextualized in the sense that its theories, concepts, methods, and tools have been endogenously developed in the ecological, economic, sociocultural, and familial contexts existing in Euro-American societies. These local contextual factors also determine or facilitate the formation and manifestation of Western people's mind and behavior for which the IP knowledge system has been established.
5. The indigenous psychological research must be conducted in such a way that the researcher's theory, concepts, methods, tools, and findings sufficiently reflect, represent, and reveal the natural structure and process of the studied local psychological or behavioral phenomenon as embedded in the socio cultural context.
6. The primary purpose for psychologists to establish a knowledge system is to interpret, understand, predict, and change people's minds and behavior such that personal adjustment can be improved and social problems prevented or solved.

As we can see, IP provides a new and different perspective from which to gain understanding of the human being. IP has multiplied the possibilities by which to the possibilities for understanding of mankind. In addition, the premise underlying IP, i.e., that it, as well as all other approaches to psychology, is rooted in and relative to its cultural background, poses a significant challenge to WP's traditional self-image of being neutral and objective. By perceiving itself as a culturally dependent, locally originated indigenous psychology, WP may achieve a more realistic self-image.

The concepts presented in this chapter make it evident that professionals who work in collaboration with parents of children with disabilities must be equipped with a broad understanding of the indigenous population and of the necessity to adjust their work methods according to this information. In this context, it is hard to imagine effective collaboration without awareness of the indigenous culture, familiarity with the dual significance of lands and territories as well as with other aspects of indigenous knowledge, and comprehension of indigenous psychology.

References

Anderson, J., & Kirkham, R. (1999). Discourses on health: A critical perspective. In H. Coward & P. Ratanakul (Eds.), *A cross-cultural dialogue on health care ethics* (pp. 47–67). Waterloo, ON: Wilfred Laurier University Press.

Ardila, R. (1982). Psychology in Latin America today. *Annual Review of Psychology, 33*, 103–122.

Azuma, H. (1984). Psychology in a non-Western country. *International Journal of Psychology, 19*, 145–155.

Azuma, H. (1988, August 28–September 2). *Are Japanese really that different? The concept of development as a key for transformation*. Invited address at the 24th International Congress of Psychology, Sydney, Australia.

Bandura, A. (1997). *Self-efficacy: The exercise of control*. New York: Freeman.

Berry, J. W. (1974). Canadian psychology: Some social and applied emphasis. *Canadian Psychologist, 15*, 132–139.

Bohannan, P. (1989). *Justice and judgment among the Tiv*. Prospect Heights, IL: Waveland Publishing.

Burnet, A. (1980). *An introduction to ancient philosophy*. London: Methuen.

Castree, N. (2004). Differential geographies: Place' indigenous rights and local resources. *Political Geography, 23*(3), 133–167.

Choi, S. C., & Kim, K. (2003). A conceptual exploration of the Korean self in comparison with the western self. In K. S. Yang, K. K. Hwang, P. B. Pederson, & I. Daibo (Eds.), *Progress in Asian social psychology: Conceptual and empirical contributions* (pp. 29–42). Westport, CO: Praeger.

Christie, C. J. (2001). Consideration of the effect of nutritional status and disease patterns on the work output amongst Black South African workers involved in manual materials handling (MMH) tasks. *Ergonomics Society of South Africa, 13*(1), 23.32.

Church, A. T., & Katigbak, M. S. (2002). Indigenization of psychology in the Philippines. *International Journal of Psychology, 37*(3), 129–148.

Classen, C. (1999). Other ways to wisdom: Learning through the senses across cultures. *International Review of Education, 53*(3/4), 269–280.

Colombi, B. J. (2012). Salmon and the adaptive capacity of Nimiipuu (Nez Perce) culture to cope with change. *American Indian Quarterly, 36*(1), 75–97.

Dai, L. T. (1956). Japanese language as an expression of Japanese psychology. *Western Speech, 20*, 90–96.

Davis-McFarland, E., & Dowell, B. (2000). Sociocultural issues in assessment and intervention. In L. Watson, E. Crais, & T. Layton (Eds.), *Handbook of early language impairment in children: Assessment and treatment* (pp. 73–110). San Diego, CA: Delmar Thompson Learning.

Diaz-Guerrero, R. (1977). A Mexican psychology. *American Psychologist, 32*, 934–944.

Dickason, O. P. (1984). *The myths of the savage*. Edmonton: University of Alberta.

Dizmang, L. H. (1968). *Observations on suicidal behavior among the Shoshone-Bannock Indians*. Paper presented at the First Annual National Conference on sociology, Chicago.

Durojaiye, M. O. A. (1993). Indigenous psychology in Africa: The search for meaning. In U. Kim & J. Berry (Eds.), *Indigenous psychologies: Research and experience in cultural context* (pp. 211–220). Newbury Park, CA: Sage.

Eddey, G. E., & Robey, K. L. (2005). Considering the culture of disability in cultural competence education. *Academic Medicine, 80*, 706–712.

Enriquez, V. G. (1993). Developing a Filipino psychological. In U. Kim & J. W. Berry (Eds.), *Indigenous psychologies: Research and experience in cultural context* (pp. 152–169). Newbury Park, CA: Sage.

Giger, J. N., & Davidhizar, R. E. (2004). *Transcultural nursing: Assessment and intervention* (4th ed.). St. Louis: Mosby.

Graumann, C. F. (1972). The state of psychology, I. *International Journal of Psychology, 7*, 123–134.

Hader, H., Rash, J., Holyk, T., Joverl, E., & Harder, K. (2012). Indigenous youth suicide: A systematic review of the literature. *A Journal of Aboriginal and Indigenous Community Health, 10*(1), 125–142.

Hague, R., & Harrop, M. (2001). *Comparative government and politics: An introduction*. Basingstoke: Palgrave Press.

Heider, F. (1958). *The psychology of interpersonal relations*. New York: Wiley.

Henry, F., Tator, C., Mattis, W., & Rees, T. (1995). *The colour of democracy: Racism in Canadian society*. Toronto: Harcourt Brace.

Ho, D. Y. F. (1976). On the concept of face. *American Journal of Sociology, 81*, 867–884.

Ho, D. Y. F. (1982). Asian concepts in behavioral science. *Psychologia, 25*, 228–235.

Ho, D. Y. F. (1998). Indigenous psychologies: Asian perspectives. *Journal of Cross-Cultural Psychology, 29*(1), 88–103.

Ho, D. Y. F., Peng, S.-Q., Lai, A. C., & Chan, S.-F. F. (2001). Indigenization and beyond: Methodological relationalism in the study of personality across cultural traditions. *Journal of Personality, 69*(6), 925–953.

Hwang, K. K. (2010). Way to capture theory of indigenous psychology. *India Psychology Studies., 55*(2), 96–100.

Ivison, D., Patton P., & Sanders, W. (Eds.). (2000). *Political theory and the rights of indigenous peoples*. Cambridge: Cambridge University Press.

Kagitcibasi, C. (1984). Socialization in traditional society: A challenge to psychology. *International Journal of Psychology, 19*, 145–157.

Kiev, A. (1964). *Magic, faith and healing: Studies in primitive psychiatry today*. New York: Free Press.

Kim, U., & Berry, J. W. (1993). *Indigenous psychology: Experience and research in cultural context*. Newbury Park, CA: Sage.

Kim, U., Yang, K., & Hwang, K. (Eds.). (2006). *Indigenous and cultural psychology understanding people in context*. New York: Springer.

Kleinman, A. (1980). *Patients and healers in context of culture*. Berkeley: University of California Press.

LaFromboise, T., & Lewis, H. (2008). The Zuni life skills development program: A school/community-based suicide prevention intervention. *Suicide and Life-Threatening Behavior, 38*(3), 343–353.

Lynch, F. (1973). Social acceptance reconsidered. In F. Lynch & A. De Guzman II (Eds.), *Four readings on Philippine values* (pp. 1–68). Quezon: Ateneode Manila University Press.

Lynch, E. W., & Hanson, M. J. (1998). *Developing cross-cultural competence: A guide for working with children and their families*. Baltimore: Brookes.

Lynch, E. W., & Hanson, M. J. (2004). *Developing cross-cultural competence: A guide for working with children and their families* (3rd ed.). Baltimore: Brookes.

McIntosh, J., & Santos, J. (1981). Suicide among Native Americans: A compilation of findings. *Omega: Journal of Death and Dying, 11*(4), 303–316.

Mezzich, J. E., Kleinman, A., Fabrega, H., & Parron, D. L. (Eds.). (1996). *Culture and psychiatric diagnosis: A DSM-IV perspective*. Washington, DC: American Psychiatric Press.

Miller, M. (1979). Suicides on a southwestern American Indian reservation. *White Cloud Journal, 1*(3), 14–18.

Miller, S. I., & Schoenfeld, L. S. (1971). Suicide attempt patterns among the Navajo Indians. *International Journal of Social Psychiatry, 17*, 189–193.

Mink, I. T. (1997). Studying culturally diverse families of children with mental retardation. *International Review of Research in Mental Retardation, 20*, 75–98.

Moghaddam, F. M. (1987). Psychology in the three worlds: As reflected by the crisis in social psychology and the move toward indigenous third world psychology. *American Psychologist, 35*, 912–920.

Moore, C. A. (1967). *The Chinese mind: Essentials of Chinese philosophy and culture*. Honolulu: The University Press of Hawaii.

Moscovici, S. (1972). Society and theory in social psychology. In J. Israel & H. Tajfel (Eds.), *The context of social psychology*. London: Academic.

Nietzen, R. (2003). *The origins of Indigenism, human rights ant the politics of identity*. Berkeley: University of California Press.

Novins, D. Beals, J. Roberts, R. Manson, S. (1999). Factors associated with suicide ideation among American Indian adolescents: Does culture matter? *Suicide and Life-Threatening Behavior, 29,* 332–346.

Nsamenang, A. B. (1995). Factors influencing the development of psychology in Sub-Saharan Africa. *International Journal of Psychology, 30,* 729–738.

Nsamenang, A. B. (2000). Issues in indigenous approaches to developmental research in Sub-Sahara Africa. *International society for the study of behavioral developmental newsletter,* Number 1 Serial No. 38, 1–2.

Ong, C. K., et al. (2005). *WHO global atlas of traditional, complementary, and alternative medicine.* Kobe: World Health Organization.

Patel, V. (1995). Spiritual distress: An indigenous model of non psychotic mental illness in primary care in Harare, Zimbabwe. *Acta Psychiatrica Scandinavica, 92,* 103–107.

Pe-Pua, R. (2006). From decolonizing psychology to the development of a cross-indigenous perspective in methodology: The Philippine experience. In U. Kim, K. S. Yang, & K. K. Hwang (Eds.), *Indigenous and cultural Chang Gung journal of humanities and social sciences. Understanding people in context* (pp. 109–137). New York: Springer.

Poonwassie, A., & Charter, A. (2005). Aboriginal worldview of healing: Inclusion, blending, and bridging. In R. Moodley, & W. West (Eds.), *Multicultural Aspects of Counseling and Psychotherapy Series 22: Integrating traditional healing practices into counseling and psychotherapy. Pp 15–26.* Thousant Oaks, CA: Sage Publications.

Redfield, R. (1956). *Peasant society and culture: An anthropological approach to civilization.* Chicago: University of Chicago Press.

Rehm, R. S. (1999). Family culture and chronic conditions. In P. L. Jackson & J. A. Vessey (Eds.), *Primary care of the child with a chronic condition* (3rd ed., pp. 66–82). St Louis: Mosby.

Rice, B. (2003). Articulating Aboriginal paradigms: Implications for aboriginal social work practice. *Native Social Work Journal, 5,* 87–97.

Scheinin, M. (2004, April 28). Indigenous peoples' land rights under the international covenant on civil and political right. *Torkel Oppsahls minneseminar.* Norwegian Center for Human Rights, University of Oslo.

Shams, M. (2002). Issues in the study of indigenous psychologies: Historical perspectives, cultural interdependence, and institutional regulations. *Asian Journal of Social Psychology, 5,* 79–91.

Shweder, R. A. (1991). *Thinking through cultures-expeditions in cultural psychology.* Cambridge: Harvard University Press.

Sinha, D. (1984). Psychology in the context of third world development. *International Journal of Psychology, 19,* 17–29.

Sinha, I. B. P. (2003). Trends toward indigenization of psychology in India. In K. S. Yang, K. K. Hwang, P. B. Pedersen, & I. Daibo (Eds.), *Progress in Asian social psychology: Conceptual and empirical contributions* (pp. 11–27). Westport, CO: Praeger.

Slaughter, D. T., Nakagwa, K., Takanishi, R., & Johnson, D. J. (1990). Toward cultural/ecological perspectives on schooling and achievement in African- and Asian-American children. *Child Development, 61*(2), 363–383.

Smedslund, J. (1984). The invisible obvious: Culture in psychology. In K. M. J. Lagerspetz & P. Niemi (Eds.), *Psychology in the 1990's.* Amsterdam: North-Holland.

Sotnik, P., & Jezewski, A. M. (2005). Culture and the disability services. In H. J. Stone (Ed.), *Culture and disability: Providing culturally competence services.* Thousand Oaks, CA: Sage.

St Clair, A., & McKenry, L. (1999). Preparing culturally competent practitioners. *Journal of Nursing Education, 38,* 228–234.

Talor, j.(1871). *Primitive Culture. V1.*

Tsosie, R. (2001). Land, culture and community: Envisioning Native American sovereignty and national identity in the 21st century. *Hagar, 2*(2), 183–200.

Tzfadia, E., & Roded, B. (2010). *Recognition and indigenous land right: The case of the rab-Bedouin in the Negev—A comparative perspective.* Beersheba: Ben-Gurion University of the Negev.

Warren, D. M., Von Liebenstein, G., & Slikkerveer, L. (1993). Networking for indigenous knowledge. *Indigenous Knowledge and Development Monitor, 1*, 24.

Webb, J. P., & Williard, W. (1975). Six American Indian patterns of suicide. In N. L. Farberow (Ed.), *Suicide in different cultures* (pp. 17–33). Baltimore: University Park Press.

Yang, K. S. (2000). Monocultural and cross-cultural indigenous approaches: The royal to the development of balanced global psychology. *Asian Journal of Social Psychology, 3*, 241–263.

Yang, K. S. (2012). Indigenous psychology, westernized psychology and indigenized psychology: A non-western psychologist's view. *Journal of Humanities and Social Sciences., 5*(1), 1–32.

Yang, K. S., & Ho, D. Y. F. (1988). The role of yuan in Chinese social life: A conceptual and empirical life. In A. C. Paranjpe, D. Y. F. Ho, & R. W. Rieber (Eds.), *Asian contributions to psychology* (pp. 263–281). New York: Praeger.

Chapter 3
School Professionals and Parents of Children with Disabilities

3.1 School Professionals

This chapter concentrates on professionals working in education systems, mainly schools and kindergartens. The special education school is an important system for students with disabilities, as it has the capacity to respond to the needs of both the child with disability and the parents, on an ecological level (i.e., addressing all of their contextual elements, such as culture, community, and environmental conditions) and on a systemic level (special education schools concentrate on the individual child's needs, rather than on groups or the entire class). In addition, schools function as a primary framework for early prevention. This chapter uses an example of a disability from the field of mental health.

The World Health Organization estimates that approximately one in five young people under the age of 18 experiences some form of developmental, emotional, or behavioral problem, and one in eight experiences a mental disorder. Research shows that half of adult mental disorders begin before the age of 14 (Kessler et al. 2005), and that early intervention can prevent and reduce more serious consequences later in life (WHO 2004). In light of this information, it is critical to expand the role of mental health professionals in schools worldwide. Schools have the potential to affect the mental health of millions of young people, as do those who work in the schools. Research indicates that programs which promote mental health are among the most effective health-promoting school efforts (Whitman et al. 2008). Clearly, schools are greatly overlooked and underutilized as a major agency in society, which could do so much more in the area of mental health promotion and prevention of disabilities. Many international agencies are playing a leadership role to move in this direction. The recent Declaration of the Consortium for Global Infant, Child and Adolescent Mental Health, for example, sponsored by the International Association for Child and Adolescent Psychiatry and Allied Professions, calls for the world to "[f]oster the development of child and adolescent mental health policy as an integral part of education, social welfare, health policy and health reform and to recognize and intervene at the earliest possible developmental stage to promote

I. Manor-Binyamini, *School-Parent Collaborations in Indigenous Communities: Providing Services for Children with Disabilities*, DOI 10.1007/978-1-4614-8984-9_3, © Springer Science+Business Media New York 2014

positive mental health and to avert the consequences of growing up with conditions which interfere with healthy mental development. Many (disabilities) can be prevented through promotion and intervention, especially through schools." The International Alliance for Child and Adolescent Mental Health and Schools, a member of this consortium, is working globally with school principals, policy makers, and researchers to promote this aim.

Due to the unique characteristics that distinguish special education schools from regular schools and other support systems, the special education school framework is able to provide an ecological, systemic, and preventive response to the needs of children with disabilities and their families. As such, it functions as an organizing framework for support services for students aged 3–21. The first part of the chapter presents the unique characteristics of these schools, followed by a description of the support services they provide. At the heart of the work of the special education school lies the conception or recognition that all children have the right to learn, while accepting the differences between people as a basic and natural condition. This recognition is anchored in legislation that calls for the preservation of human dignity and equal opportunity. An advanced society takes care to develop diverse ways for making educational adjustments to ensure that students with disabilities have an equal opportunity for optimal development. This conception serves as the basis for the education, teaching, and treatment that these schools provide. It is also the principle that dictates the schools' unique characteristics, which are as follows:

(a) Special education schools have students with a wide and complex range of unique disabilities and subsequent needs. Thus, for instance, for the majority of students in these schools, the disability presents with comorbidity: autism with mental retardation, behavioral disorders with a hearing disability, and so on.
(b) Special education schools are supra-regional and serve children from many surrounding local authorities and districts. Consequently, the schools are involved and interact with many and varied community systems.
(c) Children with disabilities have rights anchored in unique legislation; abiding by these rights requires contact with and resource pooling from many government ministries, such as welfare and social services, health, social security, and other governmental departments and offices.
(d) The complexity of the children's needs requires an intensive, consistent, and unique (collaborative) work system with the children's parents.
(e) Schools work in the framework of an extended school day (usually between 8 A.M. and 5 P.M.) as well as an extended school year (no vacation except for 2 weeks in the summer).
(f) Major transitions in the life of a special education student (for example, from kindergarten to elementary school, from living at home to living in the community) have crisis-like characteristics, which require prior intervention and consistent accompaniment of the child and the immediate family.
(g) Professionals from a variety of areas work in these schools. The expertise, orientation, and responsibility of the professionals working in special education schools concern all aspects of the students' lives: emotional, social, academic, developmental, functional, behavioral, health, and family.

Due to all of these unique characteristics, special education schools are a framework that contains all the support services that students with disabilities require. The areas of expertise are diverse and vary with the needs of the school population. Thus, the professionals who most commonly provide services in these schools are affiliated with the following disciplines and domains: education, nursing, speech-language pathology, occupational and physical therapy, medicine, social work, psychology, assistive technology, health, nutritional science, respite care, special instruction, optometry and ophthalmology, and transportation (Faircloth 2006, 25).

The aforementioned cultural notion of mainstream interventionists may differ widely from those held by other cultural groups. Members of other groups may turn to elders, another family member, a friend, or to folk healers for assistance in child health and behavior issues. To illustrate differences across cultural groups, Randall-David (1989, p. 26) provided a list of therapeutic agents or people whose help is sought for psychosocial disorders (Table 3.1).

Table 3.1 Therapeutic agents across cultural groups	Mainstream White American or European	Mexican American
	Counselors	Curanderos
	Psychiatrists	
	Psychologists	Puerto Rican
	Social workers	Espiritistas
	Ministers	Santerios
	African American	Cubans
	Ministers	Santerios
	Social workers	
	Voodoo priests	
		Southeast Asian American
		Herbalists
	Native American	Family or friends
	Native medicine men	Diviners
	"Singers"	Haitian
		Voodoo priests

Thus, the parents of children with disabilities will approach the search for help, support, or intervention in a variety of ways, according to their cultural expectations and values. At times, their choices are also related to the availability—or lack—of professionals in the indigenous community. As described in the Chap. 1, some indigenous communities lack professionals in various fields. Thus, for instance, for many years, the Bedouin community in the Negev in Israel had no Arabic-speaking speech therapist.

3.1.1 The Benefits of a Multidisciplinary Team

In countries that enjoy a wide variety of professionals, the experts are all supposed to work together as a multidisciplinary team, by law (e.g., Israel). This type of team approach is even more important in indigenous communities. First, I will define the multidisciplinary team, and then I will present the arguments inherent in such a work policy.

A multidisciplinary team can be defined as a small group of professionals from different fields of expertise, working together across formal organizational boundaries in order to provide services to the pupils. Huxham says "[w]orking together with [the] other is never simple, but when collaboration is across boundaries the complications are magnified" (Huxham 1996).

Based on the unique characteristics of special education, I would like to offer the following definition of the term "multidisciplinary team." The work of the multidisciplinary team with pupils with disabilities is intended to help cope with and find applicable ways to address school level issues and problems, from simple to complicated, by integrating different fields of knowledge, as dictated by the nature of the information, the problem, or the issue at hand. These are long-term connections between experts in a number of fields producing work that leads to new ways of action with synergetic results, beyond those common in actions deriving from separate fields of knowledge or from links between fields. This approach integrates processes of action and processes of learning and leads to the empowerment of individuals and groups, resulting in effective measures that advance the pupils with disabilities and their parents.

The rationale for applying the multidisciplinary approach as a policy contains eight major arguments (for the eight arguments, see Manor-Binyamini 2011a). Here I present only three of the eight that are relevant to schools working with parents in indigenous communities and another argument uniquely related to multidisciplinary teams working in indigenous communities.

(a) The most common argument in favor of a multidisciplinary team is based on the fact that solutions to complex problems require a wide spectrum of knowledge and abilities (Heinemann 2002; Payne 2000). More specifically, responding to the unique needs of a pupil with complex and/or multiple disabilities in a school for special education requires expertise in more than one field of knowledge: in an education system, this can be achieved only by efficient team work. Multidisciplinary work can enable a new and different look at the situation and also the identification of new opportunities for action (Lasker and Weiss 2003). Moreover, combining ideas and professional approaches in ways never before attempted may lead to new breakthroughs.

(b) A variety of professional abilities and the sharing of knowledge are considered necessary conditions for viewing the pupil holistically. The holistic approach to the pupils means considering the individual's needs from multiple perspectives, including developmental, academic, functional, social, emotional, behavioral, and family contexts. Professionals working in one specialized field can explore one particular aspect, which renders only a partial profile of the pupil's current functioning and needs (Proctor-Childs et al. 1998). A holistic outlook is an absolute necessity when working with indigenous communities. Indeed, it would be impossible to assess and help children and their families without addressing the surrounding environment, or without taking into account the unique characteristics of the community, such as its culture, indigenous knowledge, and indigenous psychology.

(c) Another argument worth considering is that the child's learning becomes more effective if the professional team members have acquired multidisciplinary skills (Littlewood 1988). Conducting shared consultations with multiple team members affords the specialists the opportunity to broaden their knowledge base and to learn about other fields of expertise. In light of this enhanced scope of knowledge, the specialists gain a better understanding of the ways in which their particular expertise can combine with and complement that of the other team members. Multidisciplinary work in special education can be carried out in different forms and incorporate a variety of participants in a variety of fields of expertise—educators, occupational therapists, speech therapists, social workers, teachers, doctors, and psychologists.

An additional argument, which is not included in the eight general arguments for the importance of multidisciplinary teamwork, is the ability to provide an appropriately sensitive response to the needs of the children and their parents, while pooling existing resources in the indigenous community. A pertinent example concerns an officially unrecognized Bedouin village (see review in Chap. 2). Given the village's nonexistent or illegal status, no government agency (Ministry of Education, Ministry of Welfare, or Social Security) has precise data regarding the number of children with disabilities in the village.

3.2 Locating Children with Disabilities in the Bedouin Community

About half of the Bedouin community, over 70,000 people, still lives in tin tends without running water or electricity, in small tribal concentrations. This population is spread out over a large area, half of which is outside any municipal support system. Families with children with disabilities face serious problems of access, due to the lack of public transportation, the high cost of forms of transportation that are not available publically, distance of the home from the road, and traditional patterns that forbid the mother from leaving tribal grounds unattended. This situation has led, in the past 8 years, to a great disparity between the number of Bedouin children with disabilities known to government authorities and their actual number in the Negev. In practice, there are thousands of children whose families despair: the children remain near the tents, do not attend school, and do not receive any treatment. This disparity underscores the great and urgent need to locate Bedouin children with disabilities and offers them the appropriate interventions and treatments, provided by a multidisciplinary team that includes all of the professional experts serving this population.

3.2.1 The Pilot Study

The purpose of the pilot study presented here was to locate every child with a disability in the Bedouin community and evaluate the effectiveness of each phase in the

Fig. 3.1 The process of
locating children with
disabilities in the Bedouin
community. GIS—
Geographic Information
System

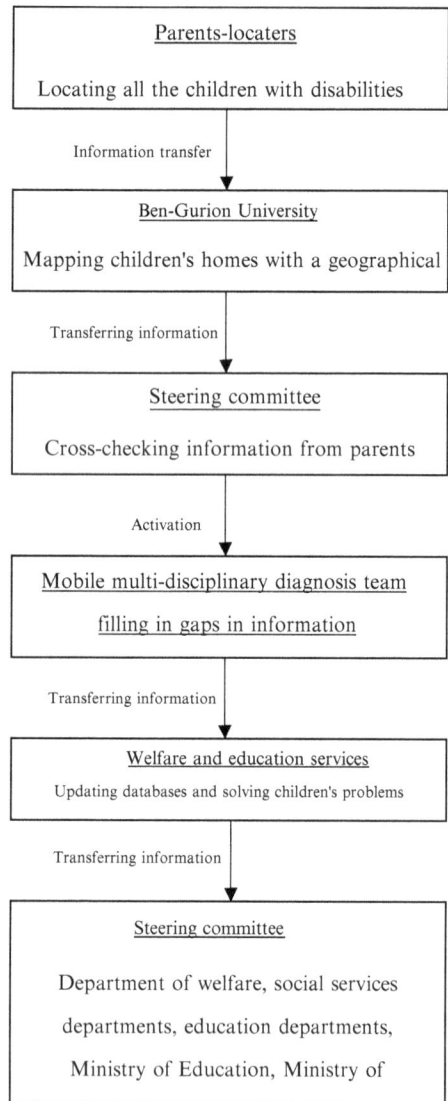

process of locating, identifying, and diagnosing children with disabilities in this
village. A unique and important component of the pilot was the participation of
parents of children with disabilities in this process. The pilot included a number of
phases, some of which were conducted concurrently and some consecutively (Manor-
Binyamini 2007) (Fig. 3.1).

The pilot study was conducted in one of the unrecognized villages in the Negev,
which had 1,000 children under the age of 18. All of the village inhabitants belonged

to one tribe and to one of six extended families. According to calculations based on a social security survey, there were supposed to be 42 children with disabilities in the community. The pilot study was conducted in 2006.

3.2.2   The Design of the Study

Phase A—Fathers of children with disabilities who were known to the social services department, were located. The fathers were asked to serve as locators in their extended family in the community. The community was divided into six "extended family sectors," with each parent/locator responsible for one sector, according to family affiliation. The parent/locators were instructed by a location coordinator (a professional working with the researcher) as to how to fulfill their role, and several simulations were conducted of cases and the possible responses they should give the parents, for instance, if a parent denies the existence of a problem with a child who is known to be disabled. In this meeting, the location coordinators received location forms and explanations on how to fill them correctly.

Phase B—A meeting was held with the location coordinator and the parents/locators in their village, and was attended also by representatives of the Steering Committee, and village dignitaries. In this phase, the purpose of the pilot study was explained.

Phase C—In 3 weeks' time, the locators surveyed the families in their sector and filled out the location forms. This activity was supervised and attended by the location coordinator, working together with a social worker assigned by the project (one social worker for each village).

Phase D—Upon concluding the location phase, meetings were held with the head of the pilot study in which each parent reported the findings in his sector and identified the homes of each located child, including those familiar to the support services, on a GIS map of the community (see Fig. 3.2).

Phase E—The data gathered by the parent/locators was cross-checked by the location coordinator and the social worker against the data in the support services' files.

Phase F—Following the discovery of 12 children who had not been known to any of the support services (welfare, education, health), the multidisciplinary mobile diagnosis team entered the field, went from one tent to another conducting diagnoses as well as social evaluations.

Phase G—Interviews were conducted with the parents of each child with disabilities in order to ascertain their needs vis-à-vis the health, education, and welfare systems.

Phase H—Workers from the Department of Welfare Services and the department of education began to work to find solutions for the problems of the newly identified children with disabilities.

Phase I—The Steering Committee held a meeting to discuss complex problems that came up during the location phase, with each government ministry representative (education, welfare, and health) taking upon himself to solve the problems in his jurisdiction.

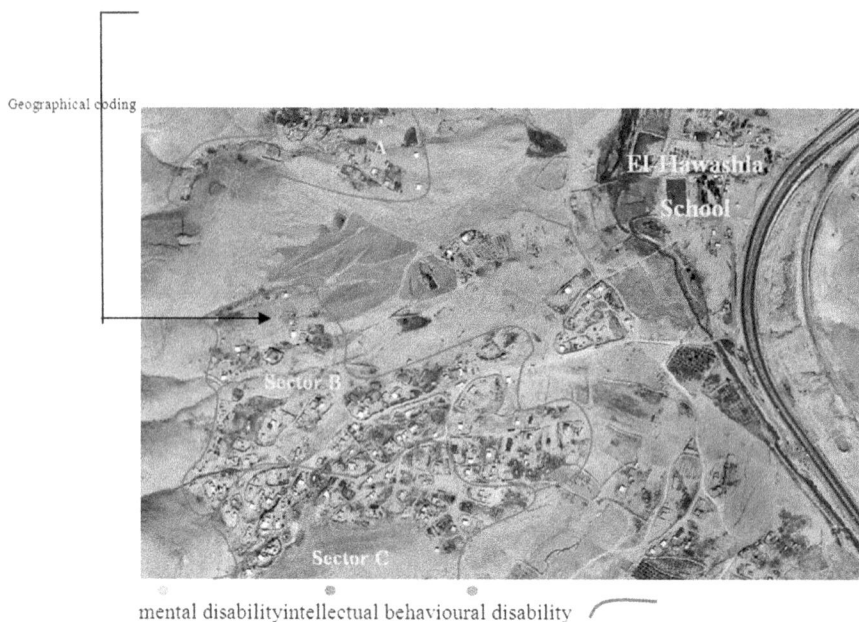

mental disabilityintellectual behavioural disability

Fig. 3.2 Picture of the social–spatial situation in the village in which the location process was conducted using geographical coding

A seminar was held with the parents/locators with the purpose of forming a group of activists to help improve the conditions of children with disabilities in the village.

3.2.3 Results

All in all, *54 children and youths* with disabilities were identified in the location and diagnosis process. Of the 54 children, 22 were diagnosed with intellectual disability (4 severe, 6 moderate, 12 light to moderate); 24 were diagnosed with multiple disabilities; 6 with intellectual disability; 13 with cerebral palsy; 5 with behavioral disorders; 3 sensory disabilities; and 5 children were diagnosed with mental disorders.

Of the 54 children, 12 children were diagnosed for the first time, as a result of the pilot study.

ID number	First name	Surname	Sex	Date of birth	Disability	Educational framework
xxxxxxxx-x	aaaa	zzzzzzz	M	20.12.95	Intellectual disability	El-Hanan school
xxxxxxxx-x	bbbb	mmmm	F	01.04.04	Behavioral disorder	None
xxxxxxxx-x	cccc	nnnnnn	F	13.04.99	Cerebral palsy	None
xxxxxxxx-x	dddd	yyyyyy	F	05.09.00	Mental disorders	El-Hanan school
xxxxxxxx-x	eeeee	kkkkkkk	M	31.07.88	Moderate intellectual disability	None

3.3   The Parents

Why do multidisciplinary teams in special education schools work with parents consistently and constantly (contrary to other areas of expertise such as social worker that work with all the family). The answer is that parents are the experts on their children, and professionals need to listen carefully to what they have to say (Coonrod and Stone 2004). For example, a growing body of literature suggests that parental reports of ongoing behavior are as accurate as test results (Goin and Myers 2004; Oliver et al. 2002).

Due to their daily interactions with their children, parents are the primary source of information, as well as the most influential figure in the life of the child; consequently, the manner in which they carry out their role has a significant, direct and indirect effect both on the etiology of the disorder and on the treatment of their children. For example, parents have both a direct and an indirect effect on the adolescent child's behaviors. The direct effect is disrupted and chaotic; in fact, studies have shown that coercive parenting covaries with levels of antisocial behavior in preschool (Shaw et al. 1996) and in childhood (Patterson et al. 1992). Parenting seems to have an indirect effect on modulating at-risk youth involvement and exposure to deviant peers, by virtue of the role of parent management, in general, and parent monitoring, in particular (Dishion and McMahon 1998). Parents provide invaluable insights into their child's social situation (Spiegle and Vandenpol 1993), and offer a context in which meanings can be attached to the child's experiences and actions, demonstrating issues pertinent to the disabled child (Brown 1998). In the case of children who are completely (or for the most part) unable to communicate (due to incapacity or age), parents hold the key to accessing the children's personal experiences and background.

Thus, professionals ascribe immense importance to the parents as sources of information and influence, as well as to the manner in which the parenting of children is conducted. The latter is the focus of the next section.

3.3.1   Children with Disabilities and the Act of Parenting

Parenting is a multifaceted phenomenon. Parenting has long been referred to by artists as a rich sequence of significant experiences that alter and shape the world of the adult. By contrast, developmental and clinical psychology, which also recognizes parenting as one of many stages in the development of man, has referred to it mainly as a role that sustains the family institution and especially the socialization of children. However, in recent years there has been an apparent change, expressed in clinical, experimental, and theoretical studies, which have begun referring to parenting as a rich internal experience as well as a significant interpersonal one. It appears that this experience raises strong and complex feelings, involves new thought processes, and activates important developmental processes.

As a role, parenting has exceptional characteristics that distinguish it from all other roles that people fulfill in adulthood. One prominent quality is that it is based on a uniquely intensive interpersonal relationship, involving commitment, responsibility, and emotional and practical nurturing, all of which require an enormous investment unrestricted by time and place. The strong moral internalization of the importance of this role and the attendant social expectations do not permit parents the right to relinquish this responsibility, suspend it, or experience burnout.

Often, assuming the parenting role occurs without proper preparation, and role expectations are colored by cultural and contextual messages. In research, most studies have focused on the influence of parents on their children and only a minority on the influence of children on their parents (O'Connor 2002). In this context, several ideas regarding the significant components of the parent–child relationship have been grounded in research and are generally agreed upon (O'Connor 2002; Shonkoff and Phillips 2000). Thus, for instance, knowledge regarding the importance of the quality of attachment between parent and child in infancy, based on the consistency, availability, and sensitivity of the parent's response to the infant's signals, needs, and lifelong socioemotional development has received much support (Sroufe 2005). The advantages of an authoritative style of parenting have also come up in many studies, which show that displaying affection and parental involvement, utilizing encouragement and positive reinforcement, active monitoring of children's activities, and consistent—though not tough—discipline, are linked to children's psychosocial adaptation measures, including academic competence, a strong feeling of self-worth, positive social relations, and few behavioral problems (Gray and Steinberg 1999).

Currently there is no single, clear, general, agreed upon theory of parenting (O'Connor 2002). In the absence of such a theory, most of the knowledge accumulated today is discrete, and describes links between various expressions of parenting and unique results among children, while raising hypotheses regarding the mechanisms involved in these effects. As a result, an attempt to digest all the information in the five thick volumes of the Handbook of Parenting, edited by Bornstein (2002), can be overwhelming, making it evident that our knowledge concerning the complexity of the issues involved in parenting is still fragmentary. One of the missing fragments concerns the parenting of children with disabilities in indigenous communities.

Giving birth to and raising a child with disabilities is a continuous care experience, which requires parents to adopt new and unfamiliar life patterns, different from those followed by others in their environment. Researchers have studied families and parents of children with disabilities for at least 4 decades, and they continue to add new reports at a high rate. These studies are often eclectic in choice of questions, variegated in methods, and protean in scope. As a collection, the research has cast light on important aspects of immensely complex phenomena. Disabilities occur in every nation, with parents often providing lifelong care to their affected child. Most research into family/parent caregiving has been undertaken in Western, English-speaking societies. Lately, there has been a growing interest in cultural differences within countries; yet, to date, there is a relative paucity of research in indigenous communities.

Research shows that for many families, having a child with a disability adds stressors to the parenting role and affects the family dynamics as a whole. The parents of these children have to confront a variety of issues in several domains of life, among them, economic, personal, couple, parenting, and social difficulties. Given that such constraints and changes are likely to add to the regular stresses of raising a child (Gallimore et al. 1999), they may lead to parental burnout, as well as physical and mental exhaustion (Lazovsky 1999).

These difficulties can bring about changes in the family and violate an existing, balanced family pattern and may especially change the parents' reaction to their child and the disability. I will present the main models found in the research literature, which detail the parents' responses to giving birth to and raising a child with a disability. Since all the models presented have been examined and constructed in the West, I will refer to or emphasize at the end of each aspect related to indigenous communities.

3.3.2   Psychological Models of Parents' Reactions

"Several psychological theories have been posited to explain parental reactions to the "news" of a disability diagnosed in their child" (Dale 1996). Although these cannot fully explain the full range and intensity of parental reaction, they offer useful guides and ideas for practice. Models offer either a "personal" (parental adjustment is a problem within the parent or individual) or "interpersonal" (adjustment has a social dimension) perspective on adjustment to disability, and both have implications for professional intervention.

3.3.2.1   Stage Model

Parents pass through a series of emotional stages before accepting, for example, a diagnosis (review by Blacher 1984). Drotar et al. (1975) defined these stages as shock, denial, anger/sadness, adaptation, and reorganization. The stage model focuses upon these emotional adjustments following the diagnosis. This reduces the chance of parental reactions being perceived as inappropriate or pathological. The notion of sequences of stages allows for appropriate and timely professional intervention (Dale 1996). However, the stage model also implies right or wrong adjustment, suggesting that deviation from the sequence is psychopathological (denying the disability). The model is methodologically weak in that not all parents go through the stages in that particular order; parents can go through more than one stage at once, can miss a stage, and may experience relief instead of grief (Blacher 1984). Furthermore, we do not know whether parents of children with disabilities in indigenous communities experience some or all of the reactions presented above. Therefore it is important to examine whether some or all of these reactions can indeed be found among parents in indigenous communities.

3.3.2.2 Personal Construct Model

Cunningham and Davis (1985) focused on cognitive interpretations of disability, rather than on emotional reactions. Parents experience different reactions because they bring different interpretations to the situation. These interpretations stem from their previous expectations of themselves and of their child. The model derives from Kelly's (1995) theory of personal constructs, which suggests that people construct models in order to anticipate events. The assumption is that people want to anticipate what happens to them and to those around them. An advantage of this model is that parents are seen as individuals with their own perspectives. This is crucial for partnership work, as it allows professionals to accept the reality of their (parents') interpretations. Personal Construct Theory has been very influential in the development of the Negotiating Model (Dale 1996). It recognizes multiple perspectives and individual diversity, constructing development as a dynamic process of internal organization, external experiences, and interactions with others. Consequently, certain experiences might facilitate or undermine adjustment, and adaptation to disability is relative to the parents' situation at the time. However, Cunningham and Davis (1985) failed to address possible unconscious determinants of behavior (cf. psychoanalytic theory) and neglects emotions (Dale 1996). Based on this model, it is important to understand, examine, and be dynamically aware of the parent's interpretation of the disability. This is an important point, especially in indigenous communities, since the parents' interpretation is based also on culture, indigenous knowledge, and indigenous psychology (for more information on these terms, see Chap. 2).

3.3.2.3 Meaninglessness and Powerlessness

Seligman and Darling (1989) considered beliefs, values, and knowledge to be socially determined through interactions. The news of a disability in the family prompts parents to "take the role of the other" in order to understand the meanings that others attach to the situation. Thus, the parents attach meanings to their experience as a result of definitions encountered in interactions with others, especially significant others (friends, family). In other words, the manner in which others define a given situation influences the parents' definition of their own situation. In this sense, this model is based on social processes and interpersonal interactions. A feeling of powerlessness is often experienced by parents in the context of professionally controlled settings (e.g., hospitals) and this feeling can intensify if, for example, birth events don't meet expectations or if medical concerns are not revealed, as when members of the medical staff unintentionally convey that something is not as it should be. Staff may also deliberately withhold information, which can create a feeling of meaninglessness for parents. This uncertainty may become more stressful than the real news (Dale 1996). Powerlessness will not abate until the parents begin to actively address their child's condition.

3.3.2.4 Eclectic Approach

Dale (1996) suggests an eclectic approach to parental reactions, drawing upon the positive aspects of each psychological reaction model. She maintains that there is a need to redress the imbalance that has characterized the research regarding parents' reactions, by examining positive parental reactions to disability (Turnbull and Turnbull 1985; Byrne et al. 1988). Researchers and practitioners have tended to focus on negative and pathological parental reactions (Lecavalier et al. 2006; Tomanik et al. 2004; Weiss et al. 2003), at the cost of positive ones. Dale (1996) asserts that professionals must stop "pathologizing" parental experiences, as this upholds devaluing attitudes towards disabled people and contributes to practices of discrimination, which, in turn, leads to segregation and long-term disadvantage.

It seems that until we have accumulated sufficient research-based knowledge concerning parents' reactions to their children with disabilities in indigenous communities, professionals would do well to adopt Dale's suggestion (1996) of an eclectic approach to parental reactions, combined with the newer approaches that emphasize stress and coping.

3.3.3 The Stress and Coping Approach

There is extensive evidence that parents of people with disabilities are at increased risk of experiencing elevated levels of stress (Blacher and Hatton 2007; Emerson et al. 2006). Therefore, research has centered on developing a theoretical representation of how families adapt to the potentially stressful situation of having a child with a disability. With this focus, researchers have steadily refined and elaborated the classic ABCX model, originally developed by Reuben Hill (1958). Essentially, this model describes "family crisis" (X) as an interactive outcome of three factors: (a) an initial stressor event, combined with (b), a family's resources for dealing with crises, and (c) the family's definition of the stressor (Behr et al. 1992; Patterson 1993). Over the last few years, the use of this and other models of family coping and resilience has allowed researchers to increasingly recognize and interpret the many successful coping strategies and positive adaptations that many families report (Manor-Binyamini 2012a, b).

Nowadays, most of the more recent research on family stress aims to identify the factors that contribute to successful coping, as demonstrated by some of the parents. Specifically, the focus now is on understanding the factors associated with the amelioration of the "crisis" (see for example research on mothers in indigenous communities, Manor-Binyamini 2011b).

Despite the increased interest in family research over the last decade, there is still a need for more extensive research on parents, reflecting on the full range of details in the daily life and routines of parents (and the family). A continuing gap in our knowledge of parents/families and disability is related also to the neglect of cultural and generational variables.

Until recently, most research on parents/families of children with disabilities tended to gloss over the situational complexities and cultural variables that surround all of us, in the interest of making global claims about the inevitable—and always negative—responses of parents to having a child with a disability. One of the results of this emphasis has been—until very recently—complete disregard of non-European cultures. Important studies of the double minority status of being non-White and disabled have begun to appear recently (see for example, Kalyanpur and Rao 1991). The need is still immense, however, for multicultural studies that explore the diversity in the experience of disability.

Such research should enable us to understand the ways in which context and culture influence and shape parents' reliance on and experience of educational systems when their children have disabilities.

A recent shift in the research literature on parental reactions to a child's disability has led to the examination of parental coping from a new perspective, specifically, from a perception of parental coping as an inevitable condition of crisis, stress, and pathology, to recognizing that multiple, varied, and possibly positive ways of coping can serve as a valuable strategy (Blacher et al. 2005). Positive changes in the parents' lives (Scorgie and Sobsey 2000), successful coping strategies (Hastings et al. 2005), and family strength and resilience (Poehlmann et al. 2005) are considered assets. In other words, coping is no longer viewed as merely adaptive, but rather as a positive influence on the family system and a potentially valuable factor in improving support systems (Hatton and Emerson 2003). Studies that have examined parental coping from this perspective found positive results in the dimensions of personal growth, closer relationships among family members, a deeper understanding of the needs of others, more meaningful personal and social connections, and a greater emphasis on expanding social activities (Scorgie and Sobsey 2000). These results suggest that despite the difficulty of making the required changes and the pain of seeing their child's condition, many parents—and families—succeed in coping well with the difficulty of raising a child with a disability, and manage to carry on with their lives. Findings of such successful coping raise the question as to what characterizes these parents and enables them to adapt to a positive perception of their situation.

The answer is that they have been able to gather and utilize both personal resources (for example, sense of coherence, personal growth, hope) and environmental resources (such as family and community support, as well as professional support services).

Disability is also a sociocultural phenomenon. Therefore the question how parents define their child's disability and react to it is an important one when dealing with indigenous communities. Hence, also sociocultural researchers have turned their attention to parents and their experiences of raising a child with disabilities. These studies vary in terms of the focus of their investigations, the disciplinary perspectives, and their theoretical orientations, but they share an interest in how cultural meanings and social institutions shape a parent's identity and the experience of disability. The following is a summary of trends in sociocultural research on the parenting of children with disabilities.

(a) One trend has been to explore the beliefs about disability, health, and healing which are widely shared by members of a society and that guide the parents' understandings and behaviors (Quinn and Holland 1987), i.e., the cultural models of child rearing and child development which guide parenting behaviors, as well as parents' expectations and evaluations of what constitutes normal development (Weisner et al. 2005; Daley 2004; Whitmarsh et al. 2007).

(b) Another trend examines family ecologies and sustainable routines of children and youths with disabilities and those of their families. These studies examine disability and adaptation to it from the point of view of the family, parents, and children. They employ a holistic and contextual perspective as they consider adaptations in various settings over the course of childhood and youth, and focus on the real circumstances that characterize the lives of both the children with disabilities and their family members (Gallimore et al. 1996; Weisner et al. 2005; Keogh et al. 2000).

(c) Yet another trend studies of the power of societal attitudes, institutions, and policies to shape parents' experiences of disability and examines the related inequities and their effects on these experiences (Skinner et al. 2005).

(d) Disability in the context of poverty is another focus in this field of research. Raising a child with a disability can be challenging for any family/parents, but conditions of poverty and limited resources often exacerbate these challenges. Recent ethnographic studies have shown that low-income families' experiences with childhood disability are influenced by the socioeconomic conditions that dictate the availability of supportive policies and disability programs (Bernheimer et al. 2003; Fox et al. 2002; Skinner et al. 2007).

(e) The relationship between race/ethnicity and disability has not been sufficiently researched. A full-scale sociocultural examination of the difference race or ethnicity makes in terms of families' experiences of disability has yet to be done. The few studies that do exist indicate that social class, education, and English language proficiency may be more important than one's racial or ethnic classification (for one such example, see Skinner et al. 2006).

A sociocultural approach to disability leads us to ask how individuals in different communities and locations come to recognize disability, how they talk about it, and how they respond to individuals who are seen as having this condition (Edgerton 1970). Whyte and Ingstad (1995) noted that a crucial area of sociocultural investigation examines the way in which constructions of disability are linked to other cultural ideas. Thus, for example, the meanings of personhood, equality, difference, and individual rights; as well as general community perceptions of gender, poverty, class, or race influence the concept and experience of disability. Similarly, understanding the manner in which social roles and self-perceptions inform and are informed by disability, and how concepts of disability can be shaped by special programs and agencies that serve persons with disabilities—these are all important questions, worthy of in-depth examination in the future.

The challenges of raising children with disability in the Western world are immense and it is difficult for people who have not lived through these experiences to truly understand them. Given that parents of children with disability in indigenous communities constitute a dual minority (indigenous and with a disability), they are considered an especially vulnerable group. Therefore, we can assume that for these parents, the difficulties of raising a child with disability create an even more immense and overwhelming challenge.

Consequently, to achieve productive collaboration between professionals and the parents of children with disabilities requires a comprehensive study of the reactions of these parents to their children and a thorough understanding of the overall significance of the parents' role.

The role of these two partners, parents and professionals, will be the focus of the next section.

3.4 The Roles of the Professionals and Parents in Special Educational Schools

A role is a collection of activities that a person engages in repeatedly and which are mutually related to activities conducted by others. A role is shaped by a combination of internal and external factors, meaning a combination of the interpersonal and intrapersonal aspects (Kats and Kahn 1978).

The roles of parents of a child with a disability are characterized by a level of complexity and intensity not found in the general population. While all parents at some time act as advocates, information seekers, spokespersons, and public educators for their sons or daughters, these roles become more crucial for parents of a child with a disability, as the child and the family become increasingly involved with a wide variety of community service providers (Minnes et al. 2003). These roles are also crucial for the achievement of desirable outcomes in various educational settings and transitions (Grove and Fisher 1999; North and Carruthers 2005), for working with therapy programmers, and for post-school outcomes for young adults with a disability (Devlieger and Trach 1999). Also professionals have a wide variety of roles to fulfill in their work with the parents. For example, Dunlap and Fox (2007, p. 278) presented a sample menu of family support options for parents of children with challenging behaviors (Table 3.2).

In a review of family support services in children's mental health treatments, Hoagwood et al. (2010) identified the following five types of service typically included in this framework.

(a) Instruction/skill development for parents: Includes parenting strategies, anger management, and stress reduction techniques. Education about child behavior and development; review of risk factors for emotional and/or behavioral problems and their potential impact; examining intervention options, child and family service systems, and other resources.

Table 3.2 Sample menu of types of support sought by parents of children with challenging behaviors

Service	Description
Information diagnosis and prognosis	Providing information about disability, child development, availability of services, empirical basis for services, etc.
	Information may be provided in various formats (via meetings, written materials, videos, etc.)
Training	Delivery of instruction, daily schedules, etc. Training may be provided in group or individual contexts and in a variety of locations
Respite care	Provision of expert child care to offer breaks to parents and other family members—may be for brief periods (hours) or extended periods (days, weekends)
In-home assistance	Provision of skilled assistant who can help instruct parents on providing behavioral guidance during specific periods in the home or community
Counseling	Provision of expert counseling to address mental or emotional challenges
Planning	Assistance with planning the child's education program and schedule
Friendship	Assistance in locating and establishing friendships, often with other families who share the same kinds of child rearing circumstances
Access to social and medical services	Information and assistance in navigating needed social services to meet family's economic, housing, transportation, food, clothing, and healthcare needs

(b) Instruction/skill development for all caregivers: Coaching caregivers on effective ways to address child behaviors and/or ways to prevent the development of emotional/behavioral problems. Also addresses the issue of the caregiver's personal well-being (e.g., communication skills, problem solving strategies, crisis management, anger/anxiety/stress management skills).

(c) Emotional and affirmational support: Stresses communication and sharing among families and/or between service providers and families to promote caregiver's feelings of being affirmed, understood, and appreciated.

(d) Instrumental services: Concrete services such as respite care, transportation, education, and flexible funds for emergencies.

(e) Advocacy: Includes provision of information about parental rights (e.g., legislation, entitlements) and resources; skill building to help the parents advocate for services for their child; coaching on ways to effectively negotiate for services, or provision of direct advocacy to obtain services for caregiver or child; and leadership skill building to develop the caregiver as an advocate at the policy- and service system levels.

The following historical survey (Table 3.3) demonstrates the complexity of the parent's role and compares it with the roles of service professionals, in order to show the dramatic changes that have occurred in the last few decades in the West, of parent's roles compared to professionals in Western countries.

Table 3.3 A historical survey of parents' roles compared to those of service professionals

The model	Model characteristics	Type of power	Basic assumptions	Professionals' point of view	Parents' point of view	Results/goals of treatment
Psychotherapeutic counseling 1960–1950	Based on psychoanalytic theories, explanation, and observation (Freud)	Professionals possess the power; they define the norm due to professional knowledge Power is unequal as professionals have power over communication, resources, and outcomes	Professionals treat parents and children as "their case." Evaluation is characterized by clinical judgment Emphasis on finding the "optimal distance" in therapeutic relations	Medical model, the professional as expert Goal of interaction with the parent is to receive information for the diagnosis, no basis for collaboration	Parents often describe the diagnosis process as traumatic	The mother will arrive at the final stage of acceptance
Parent involvement/ instruction 1970–1960	The model strongly influenced by the issue of early prevention for children The family strongly influences the child's intelligence Parents are taught to be the teachers of their children A political model according to which parents are entitled to participate in decision-making concerning their children, and not just be service recipients	Professionals control communication and resources. Parents are viewed as lacking specific skills	Parents have the time and energy to be involved in their children's educational programs Parents that fulfill the role of the professional at home are not undermining their parental role	Parents participate in the planning, development, and evaluation of the IEP goal Forms the basis for the family IEP—the IFSP	Sometimes the parent does not want to assume the pedagogical role and just wants to be a parent, not a therapist	Parental involvement is for the benefit of the child's development and does not focus on family or parental outcomes

					Outcomes for the child and the family
The family in the center 1980 and onwards	Recognition that the family is at the center. The model identifies the relationships between family members and the environment and the community as factors influencing the functioning and development of the child. The goal of work in this model is to improve the quality of life of the entire family. Two elements are embedded in the model: 1. Family choice 2. Working with the family's strengths	Parents and support services empower each other to decide together what issues should be included and addressed and which resources are available and required	1. The family is a constant in the child's life, support services come and go 2. Collaboration between professionals and parents is possible at all levels 3. There is a complete, authentic sharing of information with the family on an ongoing basis and in a supportive manner 4. Support services refer to the child's life continuum: infant, child, adolescent and, adult	For some professionals this transition is difficult	The professionals expected parents to be experts on their child. Families expect their knowledge to be respected. Parents report a sense of greater control and of direction and of being equal partners in work
Mutual empowerment 1990 and onwards	Definitions of empowerment in a variety of disciplines and across them. Common to all definitions: 1. Processes of work 2. Mutual empowerment in which all partners—professionals and families—develop their abilities through existing resources 3. There are three components of mutual empowerment: the family, professionals, and the context in which family and professionals operate	Power is synergic, not manipulative. Collaboration itself creates power The term "power" has changed—power is the ability to build or build up, to locate resources and abilities without taking power from someone else Power is the ability to implement things and is not controlled or managed by others	Centrality of the family Family choice as the foundation for decision-making Access to resources Participation Change in the environmental ecology to a holistic, humanistic one	Requires dialog that Bailey defined (based on Paulo Friere's theory) thus: Dialog is more than a conversation between two people, dialog is a real act of creation Authentic dialog requires respect, trust, and concern This is currently being examined in research	The model is new and innovative. The role of professionals is as enablers and collaborators more than as professionals	Synergy Creation of new solutions and resources Rise in satisfaction

The table represents a summary of a chapter by Turnbull et al. (2011)

As can be deduced from Table 3.3, in the traditional relationship model, professionals use their position and expertise to make judgments and take control (e.g., the medical, doctor–patient relationship). The parental function is limited to providing information. Parents aren't brought into the decision-making process, or necessarily consulted (about their views and feelings). Consequently, the parent is a passive "client" or "patient" who opts to defer to professional judgment, rather than be involved in a negative parent–child relationship. Powerful professionals can "inflate" the scope of their roles to unrealistic proportions. Nevertheless, over the last 60 years, there have been many changes in the parents' role, and professionals have learned to work together with the parents in order to improve outcomes for children with disabilities. Perhaps the most notable change has been the shift from services based solely on professional expertise to services that incorporate the knowledge of parents as part of coordinated planning on behalf of children. Initially, professionals were considered the true experts on the needs of children with disabilities, and parents played a secondary role. As parents began to participate more actively in planning their children's education and care, collaborative working relationships built on mutual respect and shared knowledge began to emerge.

Last 20 years, legislation about special education has dramatically affected the relationship between schools and parents of students with special education needs. This legislation regulates, or tries to regulate, the role of parents in special education schools. Thus, for example, the 1997 amendments to Individuals with Disabilities Education Act (IDEA) mandated that parents of children with disabilities have the legal right to be involved in all aspects of their children's education. The IDEA stipulates that parents must be invited to participate in meetings of their children's education teams as these teams identify and evaluate the children's needs, set educational goals, and make service delivery choices. Furthermore, parents have been identified as serving a key role in effective intervention strategies for children with disabilities (Feinberg and Vacca 2000).

The missing part in this review is a historical documentation of the roles of parents and professionals in special education schools in indigenous communities. This knowledge is rarely documented in research and, hence, we can assume that gap in our knowledge cannot be overcome. All the same, recognition of the complexity of parenting a child with disability and the entrance of researchers, who themselves may be parents of children with disabilities, into the field of study has led in recent years to a new conceptual and research agenda regarding the roles of parents and professionals, which may be suitable for indigenous communities. Specifically, this refers to attempts to better understand parenting on two levels: (a) the systemic-ecological level, which relates to the environmental forces that assist or restrict parents in their coping; (b) the intrapersonal level, which relates to inner processes of parental change and development. These inner processes pertain to the world of expectations, needs, beliefs, cognitions, ways of thought, and especially the *adjustments* parents make in order to cope with raising their disabled child.

The term "accommodations" as it applies to families of children with disabilities has been defined as "pro-active efforts of a family to adapt, exploit, counterbalance, and react to the many competing and sometimes contradictory forces in their lives" (Bernheimer et al. 1990, p. 223). Making accommodations has to do with problem solving, with redesigning parental roles and relationships, and with marshaling whatever financial, social, and emotional resources a parent might have, in order to adjust to the challenge of raising a child with a disability. Accommodations are made by families in response to children with any type of disability—mental, physical, or developmental—at any level of severity. One interesting research on accommodations is that of Maul and Singer (2009), which focused exclusively on families of children with severe developmental disability (DD).

The current study's investigation of the accommodations that families make in an effort to adapt to the needs of children with disabilities is driven by two conceptual frameworks: the resiliency theory (Patterson 2002) and the ecocultural niche theory (Bernheimer et al. 1990). These two theories propose a much needed change in terms of the way in which parents of children with disabilities are typically regarded. In light of this shift in perspective, professionals suggested a new approach to the design of interventions, namely, one which is helpful and relevant to parents' daily lives. The following issues, which the professionals involved in the new design designated as focus points, were derived from both the resilience- and the ecocultural niche theory. Here, each issue is accompanied by an example (Maul and Singer 2009, 163).

(a) Coping with behavior difficulties, for example, seeking help from behavior specialists, telling children in advance what to expect in terms of the day's schedule, making special seating arrangements, choosing appropriate locations, e.g., avoiding crowded and noisy places or the home of an unsympathetic relative.

(b) Facilitating and handling social situations, for example, by arriving to family get-togethers early so the child can "acclimate," finding a church with the stated mission of accommodating families of children with special needs.

(c) Making family fun part of the coping agenda, by finding activities that the whole family can enjoy and which are developmentally appropriate for the child, and attending events especially arranged for children with special needs.

(d) Accommodating food preferences through advanced preparation, for example, avoiding foods with textures and tastes which the child finds objectionable, serving a limited number of food items which the child is likely to eat, and encouraging the child to try a variety of foods.

(e) The issue of pets in the family, whether this means having no pets, or only certain kinds of pets (e.g., fish, birds, frogs).

(f) Ensuring the child's safety, for example, by giving a nonverbal child an identification bracelet, applying for a handicapped parking sticker, making sure sharp objects in kitchens, garages, and yards are out of the child's reach, keeping the house doors locked day and night, and hiding the keys.

(g) Nighttime arrangements, for example, establishing a night time routine, allowing the child to sleep in the same room with parents or siblings on special occasions, and allowing the child to "sleep in" on weekends.

(h) Planning television family time, by watching child-oriented programs together, having separate televisions for family members.

(i) Adjusting parents' employment conditions, for example, finding a lower-paying job that offers more scheduling flexibility, or finding a job with family-friendly policies.

Presumably, some of the adjustments are suitable for parents of children with disabilities in indigenous communities and some are not. During the case study, which will be presented in the second part of this book and which examined the conceptions and the coping strategies used by parents of children with disabilities in the Bedouin community in the Negev in Israel, parents talked about the adjustments they made in order to cope with their child in the community. Thus, for instance, parents spoke of exile and changing their place of residence in order to begin a new life, enlisting protection and patronage from the local leadership, "El-Sutra" or "El-Satr" (a metaphor in Arabic meaning: to vanish, bury, hide, conceal, cover up). Parents said that they chose not to reveal the fact that had a child with a disability and sometimes they even hid the child in a separate structure, far from the tribal living grounds. The impression formed through these observations was that in this community the concept of adjustment and the steps taken in order to adjust differed from the concept as perceived by parents raising their children in the West. (While the Western reader might not qualify the actions taken by the Bedouin parents as "adjustments," as an ethnographer, I presented the parents' responses as they were given to me in relation to their definition of the term "adjustment.") No doubt this issue merits further study, and it is important that such studies be conducted within a sociocultural framework.

Sociocultural studies examine parents within their cultural, historical, and sociopolitical contexts. This type of research can include—but is not limited to—cross-cultural comparisons. Sociocultural studies use various theories and methods, but they inevitably focus on the parents' shared understandings and practices related to disability; on parents' responses and adaptations to disability; and on the influence that larger social institutions and situations of inequity have on the way in which parents understand and experience their child's disability. Sociocultural approaches take into account community contexts that matter to parents of children with disabilities, and they examine the broader systems which define and position individuals with disabilities and their parents within society. As a whole, these studies provide a more experiential and holistic view of parents beliefs and offer new tools by which to study the parents of children with disability within and across different cultural groups. It appears that this kind of research approach may be suitable for studies of the roles of parents in indigenous societies. However, it is important to note that despite the overwhelming data in support of parent participation, researchers (Colombo 2006) have discovered that parents from cultural and linguistic minorities are often underrepresented among the ranks of parents involved in the schools. This underrepresentation has been explained away in various ways, including (a) minority parents' lack of time and energy (De Carvalho 2001), (b) their embarrassment or shyness regarding their own level of education or verbal abilities (Smich-Dudeon 1996), (c) a lack of information or understanding regarding the structure of the school and accepted channels of communication (Stewart 2008), (d) feeling unwelcomed by teachers and other school personnel (DeCastro-Ambrosetti and Cho 2005), and (e) the assumptions of teachers and administrators regarding the parents' desire or ability to help in their children's schooling (Lopez 2001). Unfortunately, these and other reasons have served as barriers to the full participation of parents and families from communities with a different cultural and linguistic identity in the school's endeavors.

Table 3.4 Key characteristics of a strengths approach (McCashen 2005)

Characteristic	Description
Respect	Rights: unconditional positive regard
Teamwork	Enabling collaboration and partnership, consultation and inclusion between clients and team members
Sharing	Information, knowledge, resources, and skills. Promoting clients' strengths to enable decision-making
Social justice	Acceptance, equality, equity, participation, and self-determination
Transparency	Having things out in the open, open information and communication

Despite the existence of such obstacles, there are also several encouraging developments for professionals and parents working in special education schools.

First, the work of Wolfendale (1999) helps move forward the discussion surrounding parental involvement. Wolfendale (1999) sets out a methodological framework that places parents in a central and powerful role as research partners. Listening to parents and considering their perspectives is a way in which professionals can support the development of educational services that are sensitive and effective and that meet the needs of a diverse group of people.

Second, until the last decade or so, the word "parent" in the research literature on disability was practically synonymous with "mother" Was this simply because mothers usually cared for their children with disabilities and were often available during the day when researchers wished to contact them, or was it because mothers were more used to handling challenging and probing questions about their child? Although most studies examining the cultural context of disability still focus on mothers, attention to the father's role in other cultures has increased.

I hope that research will continue to move beyond "main effect" models to examine both mediators and moderators, with the goal of determining how to best enhance parents adaptation to a child's disability. Evaluating the subtle and not-so-subtle shades of socioeconomic status, poverty, family, community, and culture can help improve our understanding of risk and prevention.

And finally, the research literature in the last decade shows a clear direction regarding the work and role definitions of parents and professionals. It seems that educational support services are adopting or trying to adopt a strengths-based approach to delivering services for parents, sometimes referred to as parents' support perspective. A philosophy of practice that builds on parents' competencies, supports parents' right to make their own decisions, and focuses on enhancing the strengths of parents, including cultural strengths emphasizes a partnership between parents and service providers (Raghavendra et al. 2007). The desired aim is to reinforce the parents existing capacities, build on their strengths, and facilitate parent-directed changes that are meaningful and significant. The main principles of a strengths approach are listed in Table 3.4.

It appears that the strengths approach may be a suitable framework for encouraging collaboration between professionals and parents of children and adolescents with disabilities in indigenous communities, but only if it is expanded to include the unique characteristics of indigenous communities. An example of considerations

Table 3.5 Crucial characteristics of a strengths approach used in indigenous communities

Characteristic	Description
Respect	For people's culture, indigenous knowledge, and indigenous psychology
Awareness of unique characteristics of indigenous communities	High frequency health risks, child labor, the need for more extensive support services, lack of financial resources, poverty, and subjection to acts of dispossession and spirit-breaking

that are critical for this approach to work well with clients in indigenous communities is demonstrated in Table 3.5.

The approach presented here is one of many for collaboration between parents and professionals. Considering what has been presented in the current chapter regarding professionals, parents, and their roles, the departure point of this book is that professionals working with parents in indigenous communities in general, and with parents of children with disabilities in these communities in particular, require a wide range of knowledge, skills, and principles of action, in order to achieve collaboration with parents of disabled children. Professionals need several types of knowledge: Western professional knowledge (professionals must make adjustments to the intervention strategies and principles taught during university training, which must be sensitive to the indigenous community to which the parents of the child belong); sensitivity and awareness of cultural differences and their implications for practice; and contextual knowledge. The availability of such a broad knowledge base will enable professionals, in collaboration with parents, to provide an educated, relevant, and beneficial response to the needs of the parents and their child, corresponding to their life circumstances. Professional principles based on the Western secular and liberal culture have already been addressed in the literature, as has the knowledge and awareness of cultural differences in the field of special education (for example, there are models of sensitivity and cultural competence). The materials in Western literature constitute a foundation, but they are insufficient for the professionals working in the indigenous community. Professionals need to create and construct knowledge and sometimes new roles that can address the unique characteristics of the indigenous community. The next chapter will be based on types of Western culturally sensitive knowledge, but will also attempt to add to these, presenting the components that have yet to be acknowledged in the literature and examining the way in which they affect collaboration in indigenous communities.

References

Behr, S. K., Murphy, D. L., & Summer, J. A. (1992). *User's manual: Kansas inventory of parental perceptions.* Lawrence: University of Kansas, Beach Center on Families and Disability.
Bernheimer, L. P., Gallimore, R., & Weisner, T. S. (1990). Ecocultural theory as a context for the individual family service plan. *Journal of Early Intervention, 14*, 219–233.

Bernheimer, L. B., Weisner, T. S., & Lowe, E. D. (2003). Impacts of children with troubles on working poor families: Experimental and mixed-method evidence. *Mental Retardation, 41*, 403–419.

Blacher, J. (1984). Sequential stages of parental adjustment to a birth of a child with handicaps: Fact or artifact? *Mental Retardation, 22*, 55–68.

Blacher, J., & Hatton, C. (2007). Families in context. In S. Odom, R. Horner, M. Snell, & J. Blacher (Eds.), *Handbook on developmental disabilities* (pp. 531–551). New York: Guilford Press.

Blacher, J., Neece, C. L., & Paczkowski, E. (2005). Families and intellectual disability. *Current Opinion in Psychiatry, 18*, 507–513.

Bornstein, M. H. (Ed.). (2002). *Handbook of parenting* (2nd ed., Vol. 1–5). Mahwah, NJ: Lawrence Erlbaum.

Brown, S. (1998). *The orchestrated body: An anthropology of embodiment and experience in brain injured children.* Ph.D. thesis, University of Edinburgh.

Byrne, E. A., Cunningham, C. C., & Sloper, P. (1988). *Families and their children with Down's syndrome: One feature in common.* London: Routledge.

Colombo, M. W. (2006). Building school partnership with culturally and linguistically diverse families. *Phi Delta Kappan, 88*, 314–318.

Coonrod, E. E., & Stone, W. L. (2004). Early concerns of parents of children with autistic and nonautistic disorders. *Infants and Young Children, 17*, 258–268.

Cunningham, C. C., & Davis, H. (1985). *Working with parents: Frameworks for collaboration.* Buckingham: Open University Press.

Dale, N. (1996). *Working with families of children with special needs: Partnership and practice.* London: Routledge.

Daley, T. C. (2004). From symptom recognition to diagnosis: Children with autism in India. *Sociology Science and Medicine, 58*, 1323–1335.

De Carvalho, M. E. P. (2001). Family-school interactions: Lessons from personal experience. In M. E. P. de Carvalho (Ed.), *Rethinking family-school relations: A critique of parental involvement in schooling: Socio-cultural, political, and historical studies in education* (pp. 29–42). Mahwah, NJ: Erlbaum.

DeCastro-Ambrosetti, D., & Cho, G. (2005). Do parents value education? Teachers' perceptions of minority parents. *Multicultural Education, 13*, 44–46.

Devlieger, P. J., & Trach, J. S. (1999). Mediation as a transition process: The impact on postschool employment outcomes. *Exceptional Children, 65*, 507–523.

Dishion, T. J., & McMahon, R. J. (1998). Parental monitoring and the prevention of child and adolescent problem behavior: A conceptual and empirical formulation. *Clinical Child and Family Psychology Review, 1*, 61–75.

Drotar, D., Bashiewicz, A., Irvin, A., Kennnell, J., & Klaus, M. (1975). The adaptation of parents to the birth of an infant with a congenital malformation: A hypothetical model. *Pediatrics, 55*, 710–717.

Dunlap, G., & Fox, L. (2007). Parent-professional partnerships: A valuable context for addressing challenging behaviors. *International Journal of Disability, Development and Education, 54*(3), 273–285.

Edgerton, R. B. (1970). Mental retardation in non-Western societies: Toward a cross-cultural perspective on incompetence. In H. C. Haywood (Ed.), *Social-cultural aspects of mental retardation* (pp. 523–559). New York: Appleton.

Emerson, E., Hatton, C., Llewellyn, G., Blacker, J., & Graham, H. (2006). Socio-economic position, household composition, health status and indicators of the well-being of mothers of children with and without intellectual disabilities. *Journal of Intellectual Disability Research, 50*, 862–873.

Faircloth, S. C. (2006). Early childhood education among American Indian/Alaskan native children with disabilities: Implications for research and practice. *Rural Special Education Quarterly, 25*, 25–31.

Feinberg, E., & Vacca, J. (2000). The drama and trauma of creating policies on autism: Critical issues to consider in the new millennium. *Focus on Autism and Other Developmental Disabilities, 15*, 130–138.

Fox, L., Vaughn, B. J., Wyatte, M. L., et al. (2002). We can't expect other people to understand: Family perspectives on problem behavior. *Exceptional Children, 68*, 437–450.

Gallimore, R., Bernheimer, L. P., & Weisner, T. S. (1999). Family life is more than managing crisis: Broadening the agenda of research on families adapting to childhood disability. In R. Gallimore, L. P. Bernheimer, D. L. MacMillan, D. L. Speece, & S. Vaughn (Eds.), *Developmental perspectives on children with high incidence disabilities* (pp. 55–80). Mahwah: Erlbaum.

Gallimore, R., Coots, J., Weisner, T., et al. (1996). Family responses to children with early developmental delays. II. Accommodation intensity and activity in early and middle childhood. *American Journal of Mental Retardation, 101*, 215–232.

Goin, R. P., & Myers, B. J. (2004). Characteristics of infantile autism: Moving toward earlier detection. *Focus on Autism and Other Developmental Disabilities, 19*, 5–12.

Gray, R. M., & Steinberg, L. (1999). Unpacking authoritative parenting: Reassessing a multidimensional construct. *Journal of Marriage and the Family, 61*(3), 574–587.

Grove, K. A., & Fisher, D. (1999). Entrepreneurs of meaning: Parents and the process of inclusive education. *Remedial and Special Education, 20*(4), 208–215.

Hastings, R. P., Beck, A., & Hill, C. (2005). Positive contributions made by children with an intellectual disability in the family: Mothers' and father' perceptions. *Journal of Intellectual Disabilities, 9*, 155–165.

Hatton, C., & Emerson, E. (2003). Families with a person with intellectual disabilities: Stress and impact. *Current Opinion in Psychiatry, 16*, 497–501.

Heinemann, G. D. (2002). Teams in health care settings. In G. D. Heinemann & A. M. Zeiss (Eds.), *Team performance in health care: Assessment and development*. New York: Kluwer Academic/Plenum.

Hill, R. (1958). Generic features of families under stress. *Social Casework, 49*, 139–150.

Hoagwood, K. E., Cavaleri, M., Olin, S. S., Burns, B. J., Gruttadaro, J. D., & Hughes, R. (2010). Family support in children's mental health: A review and synthesis. *Clinical Child and Family Psychology Review, 13*, 1–45.

Huxham, C. (Ed.). (1996). *Creating collaborative advantage*. London: Sage.

Kalyanpur, M., & Rao, S. S. (1991). Empowering low-income black families of handicapped children. *American Journal of Orthopsychiatry, 61*, 523–532.

Kats, D., & Kahn, R. (1978). *The social psychology of organization*. New York: Wiley.

Kelly, G. A. (1995). *The psychology of personal constructs. Vol. 1: A theory of personality. Vol. 2: Clinical diagnosis*. New York: W.W. Norton.

Keogh, B. K., Garnier, H. E., Bernheimer, L. P., et al. (2000). Models of child–family interactions for children with developmental delays: Child-driven or transactional? *American Journal of Mental Retardation, 105*, 32–46.

Kessler, R. C., Berglund, P., Demler, O., Jin, R., & Walters, E. E. (2005). Lifetime prevalence and age-of-onset distributions of DSM-IV disorders in the national comorbidity survey replication. *Archives of General Psychiatry, 62*, 593–602.

Lasker, R. D., & Weiss, E. S. (2003). Broadening participation in community problem solving: A multidisciplinary model to support collaborative practice and research. *Journal of Urban Health, 80*(1), 14–47.

Lazovsky, L. (1999). *The function of social support and religious faith in parental coping with children's disabilities*. M.A. thesis, the School of Social Work, the Hebrew University of Jerusalem (in Hebrew).

Lecavalier, L., Leone, S., & Wiltz, J. (2006). The impact of behaviour problems on caregiver stress in young people with autism spectrum disorders. *Journal of Intellectual Disability Research, 50*, 172–183.

Littlewood, M. (1988). West Derbyshire community mental health team. In R. Echlin (Ed.), *Community mental health centres/teams: Information pack*. London: GPMH.

Lopez, G. R. (2001). The value of hard work: Lessons on parent involvement from a(n) immigrant household. *Harvard Educational Review, 71*, 416–437.

Manor-Binyamini, I. (2007). *A pilot study for locating and mapping children with disabilities in the Bedouin sector*. Internal report, unpublished.

Manor-Binyamini, I. (2011a). Multi-disciplinary teamwork in special education school–ethnographic triangle. In M. Haines & A. Pearce (Eds.), *Child and school psychology*. Hauppauge, NY: Nova.

Manor-Binyamini, I. (2011b). Mothers to children with developmental disabilities in the Bedouin community in Israel. *Journal of Autism and Developmental Disabilities, 41*(5), 610–617.

Manor-Binyamini, I. (2012a). Parental coping with developmental disorders in adolescents within the ultraorthodox Jewish community in Israel. *Journal of Autism and Developmental Disorders, 42*(5), 815–826.

Manor-Binyamini, I. (2012b). Parenting children with conduct disorder in Israel: Caregiver burden and the sense of coherence. *Community Mental Health Journal, 48*(6), 781–785.

Maul, C. A., & Singer, G. H. (2009). Just good different things—Specific accommodations families make to positively adapt to their children with developmental disabilities. *Topics in Early Childhood Special Education, 29*(3), 155–170.

McCashen, W. (2005). *The strengths approach*. Bendigo: St Lukes Innovative Resources.

Minnes, P. M., Nachshen, J., & Woodford, L. M. (2003). The changing role of families. In I. Brown & M. Percy (Eds.), *Developmental disabilities in Ontario* (2nd ed., pp. 663–676). Toronto, ON: Association on Developmental Disabilities.

North, J., & Carruthers, A. (2005). Inclusion in early childhood. In P. Foreman (Ed.), *Inclusion in action* (pp. 66–99). Melbourne: Thomson.

O'Connor, T. G. (2002). Annotation: The effects' of parenting reconsidered: Findings, challenges and applications. *Journal of Child Psychology and Psychiatry, 43*(5), 555–572.

Oliver, B., Pike, A., & Plomin, R. (2002). The validity of a parent-based assessment of cognitive abilities in three-year olds. *Early Child Development and Care, 172*, 337–348.

Patterson, J. M. (1993). The role of family meanings in adaptation to chronic illness and disability. In A. P. Turnbull, J. M. Patterson, S. K. Behr, D. L. Murphy, J. G. Marquis, & M. J. Blue-Banning (Eds.), *Cognitive coping, families, and disability* (pp. 221–238). Baltimore: Paul Brookes.

Patterson, J. M. (2002). Integrating family resilience and family stress theory. *Journal of Marriage and Family, 64*, 349–360.

Patterson, G. R., Reid, J. B., & Dishion, T. J. (1992). *A social learning approach: IV. Antisocial boys*. Eugene, OR: Castalia.

Payne, M. (2000). *Teamwork in multiprofessional care*. London: MacMillan Press Ltd.

Poehlmann, J., Clements, M., Abbeduto, L., & Farsad, V. (2005). Family experiences associated with a child's diagnosis of fragile X or Down syndrome: Evidence for disruption and resilience. *Mental Retardation, 43*, 255–267.

Proctor-Childs, T., Freeman, M., & Miller, C. (1998). Vision of teamwork: The realities of an interdisciplinary approach. *British Journal of Therapy and Rehabilitation, 5*(12), 616–618. 635.

Quinn, N., & Holland, D. (1987). Culture and cognition. In D. Holland & N. Quinn (Eds.), *Cultural models in language and thought* (pp. 3–40). Cambridge: Cambridge University Press.

Raghavendra, P., Murchland, S., Bentley, M., Wake-Dyster, W., & Lyons, T. (2007). Parents' and service providers' perceptions of family-centred practice in a community-based, pediatric disability service in Australia. *Child: Care, Health and Development, 33*, 586–592.

Randall-David, E. (1989). *Strategies for working with culturally diverse communities and clients*. Washington, DC: Association for the Care of Children's Health.

Scorgie, K., & Sobsey, D. (2000). Transformational outcomes associated with parenting children who have disabilities. *Mental Retardation, 38*, 195–206.

Seligman, M., & Darling, R. B. (1989). *Ordinary families, special children: A system approach to childhood disability*. New York: Guilford Press.

Shaw, D. S., Owens, E. B., Vondra, J. I., Keenan, K., & Winslow, E. B. (1996). Early risk factors and path-ways in the development of early disruptive behavior problems. *Development and Psychopathology, 8*, 669–679.

Shonkoff, J. P., & Phillips, D. A. (Eds.). (2000). *From neurons to neighbourhoods: The science of early childhood development*. Washington, DC: National Academy Press.

Skinner, D., Lachicotte, W., & Burton, L. (2006). The difference disability makes: Managing child-hood disability, poverty, and work. In J. Henrici (Ed.), *Doing without: Women and work after welfare reform* (pp. 113–130). Tucson, AZ: University of Arizona Press.

Skinner, D., Lachicotte, W., & Burton, L. (2007). Childhood disability and poverty: How families navigate health care and coverage. In B. A. Arrighi & D. J. Maume (Eds.), *Child poverty in America today: Health and medical care* (Vol. 2, pp. 50–62). Westport, CT: Praeger.

Skinner, D., Matthews, S., & Burton, L. (2005). Combining ethnography and GIS technology to examine constructions of developmental opportunities in contexts of poverty and disability. In T. Weisner (Ed.), *Discovering successful pathways in children's development: Mixed methods in the study of child-hood and family life* (pp. 223–239). Chicago: University of Chicago Press.

Smich-Dudeon, C. (1996). *Parent involvement and the education of limited-English-proficient students*. Retrieved April 17, 2009, from http://www.ericdigests.org/pre-925/parent.html

Spiegle, J. A., & Vandenpol, R. A. (1993). *Making changes: Family voices on living with disabilities*. Cambridge: Brookline Books.

Sroufe, A. L. (2005). Attachment and development: A prospective, longitudinal study from birth to adulthood. *Attachment and Human Development, 7*(4), 349–367.

Stewart, E. B. (2008). School structural characteristics, student effort, peer associations, and parental involvement: The influence of school and individual-level factors on academic achievement. *Urban Education, 40*, 179–204.

Tomanik, S., Harris, G. E., & Hawkins, J. (2004). The relationship between behaviors exhibited by children with autism and maternal stress. *Journal of Intellectual Developmental Disability, 29*, 16–26.

Turnbull, A. P., Turbiville, V., & Turnbull, H. R. (2011). Evolution of family–professional partnerships: Collective empowerment as the model for the early twenty-first century. In J. P. Shonkoff & S. J. Meisels (Eds.), *Handbook of early childhood intervention* (2nd ed.). Cambridge: Cambridge University Press.

Turnbull, H. R., & Turnbull, A. P. (1985). *Parents speak out: Then and now*. Columbus: Charles E. Merrill Publishing.

Weisner, T. S., Matheson, C., Coots, J., et al. (2005). Sustainability of daily routines as a family outcome. In A. Maynard & M. Martini (Eds.), *Learning in cultural context: Family, peers and school* (pp. 47–74). New York: Kluwer/Plenum.

Weiss, J. A., Sullivan, A., & Diamond, T. (2003). Parent stress and adaptive functioning of individuals with developmental disabilities. *Journal on Developmental Disabilities, 10*, 129–136.

Whitman, C. V., Aldinger, C., Zhang, X. W., & Magner, E. (2008). Strategies to address mental health through schools with examples from China. *International Review of Psychiatry, 20*(3), 237–249.

Whitmarsh, I., Davis, A., Skinner, D., et al. (2007). A place for genetic uncertainty: Parents' valuing an unknown in the meaning of disease. *Social Science and Medicine, 65*, 1082–1093.

WHO. (2004). *Prevention of mental disorders: Effective interventions and policy options: Summary report*. Geneva: World Health Organization.

Whyte, S. R., & Ingstad, B. (1995). Disability and culture: An overview. In B. Ingstad & S. R. Whyte (Eds.), *Disability and culture* (pp. 3–32). Berkeley: University of California Press.

Wolfendale, S. (1999). Parents as partners in research and evaluation: Methodological and ethical issues and solutions. *British Journal of Special Education, 26*(3), 164–170. School Psychology Review, 35, 645–662.

Chapter 4
Collaboration Between Parents of Children with Disabilities and Professionals in Schools

Coming together is the beginning. Keeping together is progress. Working together is success

The value and contribution of parents' collaboration with professionals who treat their children has been the focus of a great deal of social and educational debate in the twenty-first century (Stoner et al. 2005) and it is a particularly critical issue in special education frameworks. This collaboration is undergoing a transition to a new era (Kasahara and Turnbull 2005) and the social debate reflects parents increased involvement in their children's lives, a development which is deeply rooted in democratic society. From a democratic perspective, parent collaboration attests to the implementation of the rights to equality and pluralism by democratic means, as exemplified in nonprofit organizations, support groups, and pressure groups. The activities of these groups have often paved the way for legal deliberations and legislation regarding children with disability (Stoner et al. 2005). In Israel, for example, the following laws have been passed: the Special Education Law (1988),[1] Extension of Section 7 to the Law with respect to Inclusion (1997), and the Learning Disabilities Law (2003). In the USA, legislation expanded parents' rights to include informing parents about their rights and about school policy, parent involvement in planning their children's study program, as well as free access to information granted to parents. Policy derived from this law reflects the growing recognition of the importance of collaborating with parents, based on the

---

[1] Passed in Israel in 1988, the Special Education Law consists of four parts: (1) Provides definition of terms, e.g., special education, children with special needs, institutions and auxiliary servicesfor children with special needs. (2) Describes the goals of special education. (3) Focuses on diagnosis and placement issues, and (4) Relates to special schools. Only two of the 24 sections of the Law address the parents of children with disability: Section 19, which focuses on the issue of IEP individual education programs, indicates that the child's parent will be invited to a meeting when formulating such a program. Section 20 refers to a final evaluation, specifying that at the end of the school year the parents of a child in a special education school will receive a written evaluation of their child's progress in a variety of areas.

I. Manor-Binyamini, *School-Parent Collaborations in Indigenous Communities: Providing Services for Children with Disabilities*, DOI 10.1007/978-1-4614-8984-9_4, © Springer Science+Business Media New York 2014

assumption that professionals and experts cannot provide all the information and skills required to meet the varied needs of children with disability, nor those of their parents. Indeed, increasing efforts are being invested at the system level to enhance collaboration between school, support-service specialists, and the families in designing intervention programs for disability children (Shannon and Stuart 2005; Dunst and Dempsey 2007).

The discussion surrounding this change in the framework and management of educational-therapy is based on research demonstrating that certain patterns of parent–professional interaction were crucial to building strong and effective educational experiences for children with disabilities (Stoner et al. 2005). Almost 4 decades of research "have demonstrated that parent involvement significantly contributes to improved student outcomes" (Carter 2002, p. 1). "The evidence is consistent, positive and convincing: parents have a major influence on their children's achievement in school and through life" (Henderson and Mapp 2002, p. 7). As Boyer (1995) has summarized, "The message is clear. It is simply impossible to have an island of excellence in a sea of community indifference, and when parents become school partners, the results can be consequential and enduring" (1995, p. 61). It also draws on the belief that parents' collaboration in the educational process engenders more effective results for child, parent, and family alike (Fine and Nissenbaum 2000; Stoner et al. 2005). Parents' collaboration with professionals has garnered much attention in the literature over the past 2 decades (Epstein 1993; Lynch and Hanson 1998). Research indicates that parent collaboration leads to a host of positive outcomes for children with disability (Spann et al. 2003), specifically better and faster development for the child, and enhanced quality of life for the parents. The term "quality of life" refers to reduced stress and a united family with improved relationships. Numerous studies have shown a relationship between professional support and the parents' ability to deal with pressure. Appropriate support eases tension levels experienced by parents of children with disability and enhances perceived control, competence, and confidence concerning life events. This, in turn, may have a positive influence on human behavior and functioning (Nachshen 2005; Dempsey et al. 2001), can impact the ways in which parents adapt to the fact that they have a child with a disability, and may also be a factor in strengthening family fortitude (Symon 2001).

From the point of view of the professional team, collaboration among professionals in special education is viewed as a powerful tool for helping teachers who work with students with disabilities (Cox 2005). Inherent in this call for collaboration is the recognition that planning and working together is in and of itself a powerful professional development tool.

The past decade has led also to a growing awareness of the benefits of fostering collaboration with parents. Thus, for example, early resolution of disagreements reduces the need for expensive measures such as mediation, hearings, due process, and court deliberations.

The body of literature on parent collaboration with professionals in a school framework has continued to grow. Within that literature there is a plethora of insights and recommendations for improved practice. Complementing well-known work in this area (including Friend and Cook 2009; Kalyanpur and Harry 1999 and other works), researchers have undertaken a rigorous study of the complex dynamics that take place in the interactions between schools and parents, and have published their work in a variety of outlets—some of which, unfortunately, are not open to all. Hence, the target audience, namely, educators and parents, cannot benefit from this information.

The literature on the topic of collaboration of parents of children with disabilities with professionals in the special education system has developed mainly in Western countries and is informed by a Western, secular, liberal culture, which is distinct from many other cultures around the world. In recent years, awareness of cultural and lingual differences and of the effects these differences have on the practice of the profession of special education has increased, due to both the rise in the number of students of various cultural and lingual backgrounds in schools in general, as well as an overrepresentation in special education schools of children whose cultural and/or lingual backgrounds differ from the majority. A manifestation of this increased awareness is in the recognition that collaboration between professionals (experts) and parents of children in minority communities in general and in indigenous (native) communities in particular must have a different basis than the one represented in the existing Western literature, a basis which will be outlined later in this chapter. The first part of this chapter presents a working definition of the term *collaboration*. The next part describes the characteristics of collaboration as outlined in the Western literature and considers the pros and cons of this type of collaboration with parents of children with disability at special education schools. The third part reviews examples of effective practical collaboration between professionals at special education schools and parents of children with disabilities. The last part of the chapter addresses the issue of collaboration in indigenous communities.

4.1 Definition of the Term "Collaboration"

A distinction needs to be made between terms such as partnership, involvement, and various examples of good practice, which can lead to collaboration or good working relationships. Although this terms tend to be used interchangeably, there are advantages to thinking of *collaboration* as an ideal to be worked towards, whereas various forms of working together can be regarded as desirable intermediate stages along the road to meaningful collaboration.

The term *collaboration* encompasses the complexity of the relationship between parents and school professionals and is viewed as a dynamic and interactive process in which parents draw on multiple experiences and resources to define their interactions with the school and with the school professionals.

The term *collaboration* is often understood as a process, at other times as an outcome. Cook and Friend (2010) defined it more broadly as "a style professionals select to employ based on mutual goals; parity; shared responsibility for key decisions; shared accountability for outcomes; shared resources; and the development

Increasing degree of collaboration and partnership

Informing---- Involving---- Engaging---- Leading

Fig. 4.1 Stages of progress to collaboration. Adapted from Hedeen et al. (2011, p. 1)

of trust, respect, and a sense of community" (p. 3). Research on education practices across schools led Amendt (2008) to see a continuum of collaboration. After comparing his data with that presented in the existing literature, he recognized that greater collaboration between educators and parents occurs in stages along a progression, not as a single event. Figure 4.1 shows the stages of progression on the way to collaboration.

The first stage, *informing*, represents the one-way flow of communication from the school to the students and parents. Amendt draws an important distinction between the next two stages, *involving* and *engaging*, as he explains that "involvement represents an invitation to parents to support an agenda determined by the school professionals, while engagement suggests that the school professionals, the parents, and community members (together) create the agenda, make decisions, and take actions" (Amendt 2008, p. 3). His study suggests that involvement is marked by limited trust, while engagement develops a higher degree of trust. Leading occurs when the partners have created a norm of engagement, with all partners playing appropriate leadership roles as they work towards a shared vision. Parents at a school characterized by a high level of engagement found that both parties had invested effort to create the foundation of cooperation and goodwill that allowed their relationship to accrue greater trust.

Based on the above, I am suggesting a broad definition of the collaboration between parents and professionals, which is suitable for the work that takes place in the schools of indigenous communities: collaboration as a reciprocal, contextual, and interactive process, which allows for knowledge acquisition on both sides, which are in fact the products of the encounter between the two sides—the professionals bring their expert knowledge, and the parents bring parental and indigenous knowledge, that is, knowledge of their environment, community, and culture.

Hence, collaboration is a process that honors multiple realities and life experiences and produces outcomes that reflect the knowledge constructs and value systems of those who are without power (Obiakor et al. 1999). What, then, are the characteristics of a collaboration of this nature?

4.1.1   Characteristics of Collaboration with Culturally and Linguistically Diverse Parents of Children with Disabilities at School

Western literature, as outlined at the beginning of this chapter, points to many advantages that arise from the collaboration between professionals and parents, advantages for all sides: the children, the parents, and the professionals, or as Harry (2008) emphasizes: providing adequate supports can make a tremendous difference in outcomes for parents and family members of children with disabilities (Harry 2008). This is also true when referring to Culturally and Linguistically Diverse (CLD) parents. Further study is needed in order to examine the point of view of parents in indigenous communities, so that we may learn if the advantages outlined in the existing literature also apply to parents in indigenous communities. Several studies have reported that CLD families/parents exhibit lower levels of participation than European or American families in the special education process (Harry 1992; Lynch and Stein 1987). Many researchers have discussed barriers to the participation of CLD families (Blanche 1996; Chan 1990; Harry 1992; Sontag and Schacht 1994).

There may be an assortment of reasons for the barriers depicted in the literature, for example, the lack of involvement by African American parents and families may be due to parental alienation from the school in terms of feeling out of place, experiencing real or perceived discrimination, or having a sense of estrangement when interacting with the educators of their children (Bempechat 1992). As a result, school personnel may form the misconception that African American parents are apathetic, disinterested, or indifferent to their child's education and may not work to encourage these parents to participate in school-related processes (Bloom 2001). Conversely, these parents may feel as if they don't have anything to offer the school (Thomson 2003a).

Brandon (2007) identified nine factors that serve as barriers to parent participation: (a) cultural and/or linguistic diversity, (b) economic constraints, (c) family composition, (d) parent's educational level, (e) school-home communication, (f) parent–teacher interaction, (g) school–parent interaction, (h) the child's scholastic achievements, and (i) personal constraints (e.g., lack of time, lack of transportation, lack of child care). The interaction of these barriers can be complex and create a cycle of noninvolvement in which parents retreat and educators do not engage the parents.

Another detailed list of potential barriers is presented in Table 4.1.

However, parents in indigenous communities have an array of support services available to them. For example, Begay et al. (1999) examined support systems available to Navajo parents of children with disabilities.

Table 4.2 shows the results of the study.

Harry (2008) added four main themes that can become barriers to parental participation: cross-cultural differences in understanding the meaning of disability; deficit views of CLD families; cultural conflicts in the setting of transition goals; and differential understanding of caregivers' roles in the education system (for more on each clause, see Harry 2008, pp. 378–379).

The difficulties presented affect the degree of cooperation on the part of the parents, which in turn affects parents' access to and use of support services.

Parents' isolation from or lack of connection with their child's school should be interpreted as an indication that they feel out of place and experience a sense of estrangement when interacting with the school. This isolation may cause parents to express a sense of fear, depression, and even school phobia (Epstein 1995). Parents may find such a relationship marked by inconsistencies and discontinuities in points of contact, by an acute asymmetry of power (Knox et al. 2000) or even by conflict (Williams and Robinson 2001).

Table 4.1 Barriers to parents' participation

Parents/families	Professionals	Programs
Limited English proficiency	Special education professional knowledge and sensitivity to cultural diversity	Lack of language-appropriate information-materials concerning resources, rights, and responsibilities for non-English-speaking individuals
Differences in language and dialects	Insensitivity to religious beliefs and family traditions	Shortage of trained bilingual and bicultural personnel
Interpersonal communication style differences	Professional attitudes that stereotype or blame the parent and deny parental expertise and knowledge about the child	Inflexible scheduling of conference meetings with parents
Acculturation level	Professionals' withholding of information	Lack of culturally responsive service models that systematically address relevant cultural orientations and behaviors that affect service use
Attitudes towards disability	Use of jargon	
Family knowledge and comfort with the school infrastructure		
A sense of alienation from school		
Work/time conflicts		
Transportation problems		
Logistic barriers related to income, material resources, transportation, time, and/or childcare needs		

Adapted from Zhang and Bennett (2003, p. 52)

Table 4.2 Sources of support for Navajo parents

Type of support	Percentage
Church/religious including Navajo tradition	88
Other family members	84
Grandparents	64
Friends	12
Professional	*8*
Other families with children with disabilities	4

Adapted from Begay et al. (1999, p. 84)

Advance knowledge and awareness of these barriers will help professionals constructively develop strategies to facilitate parent understanding, participation, and collaboration. The power of a special education school system to increase CLD minority parents' collaboration has been well documented (Epstein 1996; Thomson 2003b). There are several suggestions in the literature as to how to achieve this goal in special education schools. From the array of existing literature, I highlight here

(a) A suggested framework that enables special education service providers to better meet the needs of the culturally diverse children and parents they serve

Fig. 4.2 Framework for providing culturally responsive early intervention services. Adapted from Bradshaw (2013, p. 3)

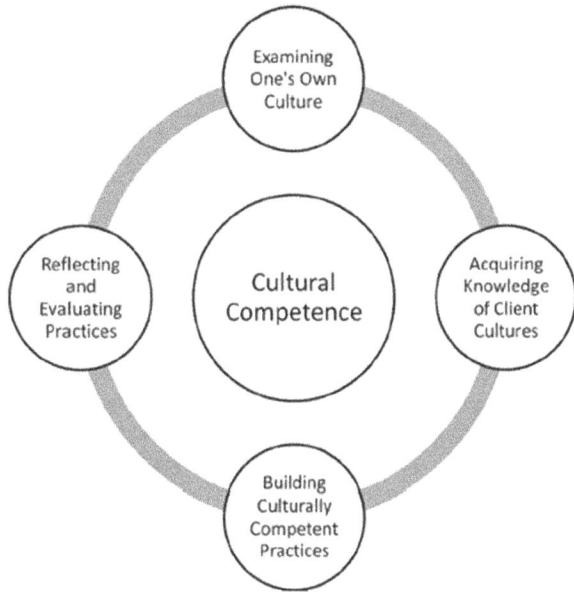

(b) Recommended strategies
(c) Traditional teachings

   (a) The framework presented here was created in an attempt to organize exist-
      ing research and literature on cultural responsiveness in a way that applies
      to the unique context of special education early intervention. This frame-
      work draws on several fields of study, including early childhood develop-
      ment, multicultural communication, special education, psychology, and
      speech-language pathology, synthesizing the knowledge and best practices
      into four guiding principles (see Fig. 4.2).

   The first principle, Examining One's Own Culture, is grounded in findings and
recommendations from experts in the fields of early childhood and special education who have all emphasized the importance of self-study for developing cultural
responsiveness and encourages professional service providers to take an in-depth
look at their own cultural values and beliefs.

   Acquiring Knowledge of Parents' Cultures highlights the importance of finding
out about the cultures of the parents/families that they serve. These first two principles serve as the foundation for the third principle, Building Culturally Responsive
Practices. This principle actively engages the provider in developing and implementing culturally responsive practices that respond to the unique strengths, needs,
and desires of parents. Finally, the fourth principle, Reflecting and Evaluating
Practices, encourages professional service providers to reflect often on their practices, so as to identify their most and least effective practices with parents of cultures
different from their own.

Table 4.3 Questions to identify underlying cultural beliefs (Bradshaw 2013, p. 7)

Overarching question	Example	Rationale
How do I communicate my respect for others?	Is eye contact important? When do I speak in a formal or informal manner?	What is considered respectful differs across cultures
What types of verbal and gestural communication are appropriate?	Do I use formal titles or conventions such as "ma'am" and "sir?"	

Several areas in which providers should examine their own beliefs in the context of their service provision have been identified. One such area concerns individual beliefs about the range considered "normal" for child development and beliefs about correcting and accepting "abnormal" behaviors (Harry 1992). Another area on which professionals should reflect is their views about what constitutes parenthood, including parents' roles and responsibilities and how enmeshed or disengaged parents should be with each other (Harry 1992).

Bradshaw (2013) also reviews some practical questions that experts should ask themselves. These questions can help them identify their underlying cultural beliefs and assumptions (Table 4.3).

The recommended strategies presented here were selected from a number of available strategies. I will describe one strategy in some detail, as an example, using Table 4.4 (for other examples, see Colombo 2006; Harry 2008; Harry and Klinger 2006; Yan and Lin 2005).

(c) *Traditional teachings* were determined based on behaviors that proved to be successful in maintaining the integrity of the indigenous community and the individual. For example, for the Native American traditional talking circle, the elements of storytelling, medicine wheel, and vision quest are the core of traditional teachings (BigFoot 1998). Traditional teachings were based on cultural values that gave essence to the traditions of Native American nations.

In addition to the frameworks, strategies, and traditional teachings, mentioned heretofore, to deal with the complexities of working with CLD parents of children with disabilities, numerous processes, and working models have been developed, which are based on several different approaches. I will outline two main approaches, both with applications in the special education system. The first, "Cultural Competence," refers to a content of multiculturalism and encourages the development intervention skills within the context of a multicultural society. The second, "Cultural sensitivity," is an approach which enables experts and professionals to develop an understanding of different cultures.

4.1.2 Cultural Competence Approach

Although there may be no universally accepted definition of the term "cultural competence," the delivery of effective support services in school to parents from various

Table 4.4 Strategies for facilitating parent/family participation in special education processes

Parents/families

  Enhance parents' knowledge and understanding of school policies, practices, and procedures

  Develop new roles for parents

Professionals

  Involve other influential family members or qualified community members

  Develop knowledge of and sensitivity for multiple dimensions of cultural diversity

  Hold bilingual meetings and select convenient times for parents

  Conduct a home visit a few days prior to Individual Education Program (IEP) meeting, to discuss with parents issues such as child care, transportation, and the importance of parent attendance

  Use family-centered approaches and collaborative techniques when interacting with families/youth with disabilities

  Understand culturally bound, nonverbal aspects of communication, such as body language and eye contact

  Reduce the volume of written information. Parents with information that is not only factual but also open-ended and reciprocal, to allow parents to express their cultural views on disability, preferences, and opinions about placement, teaching methods, and the extent and meaning of their rights under the special education law

  Provide an overview of what will take place throughout each phase of the IEP

  Orient parents to location of the IEP meeting and introduce them to other members of the interdisciplinary team

  Encourage parents to have a family member or family advocate accompany them

  Familiarize yourself with emotional reactions and attitudes to a child with a disability

  Define goals which are consistent with the life experiences, religious beliefs, and cultural values of the parents served

  Use native language information and materials (e.g., reading materials, radio, television, video, Website)

  Maintain ongoing communication regarding status of assessment and service delivery procedures

Programs

  Provide transportation, advance notice of meeting times and locations, and on-site childcare

  Hire persons who are familiar with the culture of the parents in order to promote accurate and unbiased interpretation

  Maintain the same interpreter throughout the process to avoid disruption of parent/interpreter relationship, such as churches or ethnic organizations, as opposed to impersonal efforts

Adapted from Zhang and Bennett (2003, p. 54)

cultures requires information about the specific cultures and an understanding of the ways in which culture may affect one's views of disability.

Lynch and Hanson (2004) proposed the term "cross-cultural competence," which they defined as "the ability to think, feel, and act in ways that acknowledge, respect, and build upon ethnic, sociocultural, and linguistic diversity" (p. 50).

The National Education Association (NEA 2008) has described cultural competence as the skills and knowledge needed to effectively serve students and their families/parents from diverse cultures. Four basic cultural competence skill areas were highlighted: (a) valuing diversity, (b) being culturally self-aware, (c) understanding the dynamics of cultural interactions, and (d) institutionalizing cultural knowledge and adapting to diversity. The focus here is on the internal changes an educator must go through to better teach children and interact with parents. To achieve a level of cultural competence, professionals first have to acknowledge and be sensitive to the differences among the parents with whom they work. Diller (1999) identified specific skills that educators and other school personnel should have in order to attain cultural competence. Diller suggested that educators (a) seek out educational and other training experiences to enrich their understanding and effectiveness in working with culturally different populations; (b) seek to understand themselves as racial and cultural beings and strive for a nonracist identity; (c) familiarize themselves with relevant research regarding multiracial families, (d) become actively involved with multiracial families outside of the classroom (i.e., community events, social and political functions, celebrations, friendships, neighborhood groups), so that their perspective of multiracial families is more than academic or merely a helping exercise; (e) engage in a variety of verbal and nonverbal helpful responses (i.e., they are not limited to a single method of helping, and they recognize that helping styles and approaches can be culture-bound); (f) be able to exercise institutional functions on behalf of the families; and (g) take responsibility for interacting in the language requested by the family, even if they have to seek outside persons with cultural knowledge greater than their own.

Campinha-Bacote (1999) offered a model to address cultural competence. Four constructs make up this model:

(a) Cultural awareness—The first step is becoming aware of one's own culture and the beliefs, traditions, mores, and behaviors that make up that culture. Then, the process continues with self-knowledge of one's own prejudices regarding other cultures. After understanding one's own culture and one's beliefs about other cultures, the individual gains an appreciation for other cultures as a framework with its own unique beliefs, traditions, mores, and behaviors.
(b) Cultural knowledge—The next step is cultural knowledge. After gaining an appreciation for other cultures, one must consciously seek out information and learn about the beliefs, traditions, mores, and behaviors that characterize the other culture(s).
(c) Cultural skill—Cultural skill involves further in-depth knowledge needed in order to assess, plan, intervene, and evaluate the child's education profile and status through the lens of the child's culture. In other words, the multidisciplinary team must know how to address and adapt the assessment according to the cultural beliefs and values of the target population.
(d) Cultural encounters—Cultural encounters complete the learning curve, through the experience of working professionally with children and parents from different cultures. Through this experience, professionals can become more culturally competent in their caregiving. Gaining cultural competence is a lifelong process.

The notion of cultural competence is already a well-established resource for professionals in special education. This involves open-minded willingness and training, in order to understand the situations of individual parents in light of the culture that influences their perspective (as well as the ability to recognize divergences from the parents own cultural world).

Additionally, there has been great interest in the topic of cultural competence, and so there are a number of practical applications, existing approaches, and working formats within the field of special education, which have been modified to apply to parents of different cultures. One such approach that can be outlined here is PBS—Positive Behavior Support. An emphasis on parents and families working in collaboration with professionals is a core PBS value (Lucyshyn et al. 2000). Building collaboration refers to establishing a truly respectful, trusting, and reciprocal relationship between professionals and parents, for the purpose of conducting function assessment, designing behavior support plans, and sharing responsibility for PBS implementation. Research has documented that collaboration between parents and professional is an important component that influences the effectiveness of PBS practices (Hieneman and Dunlap 2000). More specifically, informed understanding of parents and families from various cultural backgrounds is vital to the success of any intervention, including PBS (Lynch and Hanson 2004).

4.1.3 Cultural Sensitivity

There are a number of working models and/or working processes applicable to the tasks shared by parents and professionals in the special education system, which attempt to provide a solution to the cultural differences between the two parties. In regards to the "Cultural sensitivity" models, I have chosen to outline one particular procedural model, known as Biculturalization (Fong et al. 1999), which has been proven empirically to be effective when applied specifically to collaborating with families in planning an intervention or an Individual Education Program.

Biculturalization, originally used in the field of social work, is designed to create culturally appropriate interventions, by identifying and integrating the compatible beliefs and values found in a Western intervention with those of an indigenous intervention. Biculturalization can be used in special education as a process for including parents in culturally responsive IEP planning. Biculturalization was chosen as the indigenous process because it has been used effectively to build collaboration between professionals and parents. Biculturalization consists of five steps, which are presented here briefly.

1. Identify the important values in the ethnic culture which can be applicable in the merged approach
2. Choose a Western approach with a theoretical framework and values are compatible with the ethnic cultural values of the participants
3. Analyze an indigenous approach familiar to the ethnic participants, in order to determine which aspects can be reinforced and integrated into the Western approach
4. Develop a framework that can integrate the values and techniques of the ethnic culture and allows for a combination of the indigenous and Western approaches
5. Apply the Western intervention by explaining its framework and approach and how they help reinforce the indigenous cultural values and approaches (Fong et al. 1999, p. 105)

As shown, the topic of collaboration between parents and professionals is a complicated one; nevertheless, there are expert groups of interdisciplinary professionals who successfully collaborate with parents in indigenous communities. The following subchapter features an example of such effective collaboration.

4.2   Effective Collaboration Between Professionals and Parents of Children with Disabilities at Special Education Schools

The parents of an exceptional child are on an emotional journey that we, as external observers, will never be able to fully comprehend or appreciate. We can only respect this journey. (Art therapist and mother of an exceptional child)

So many words have already been written and spoken on the subject of collaboration with parents that it may be helpful to think in concrete terms about day-to-day practical ways in which parents and professionals could work together more meaningfully in special education schools.

For many years, regular and special educational settings encouraged collaboration between professionals and parents in kindergartens, schools, and development centers, for the reasons specified above. Nonetheless, research reveals an unexplained gap between the theoretical interest expressed by professionals in creating such collaboration, and the reality in the field. Despite the significant support in favor of collaboration expounded by theoretical literature in the field (Pinkus 2005; Maddock 2002; Blue-Banning et al. 2004) and the many years of legislation, research, and experience, achieving effective collaboration between parents and professionals/interdisciplinary remains a challenge.

To help address the challenge and to further clarify the nature of positive collaboration between parents and professionals, I conducted a study to examine precisely how this collaboration takes place in daily life, what the professionals do, and how parents engage. The study attempts to identify the components of effective collaboration between professionals and parents, to discuss the core components that constitute the basis for collaboration as it takes place in practice, and to consider the behavioral expressions of these components.

As collaboration also entails mutuality, the study places particular emphasis on successful collaboration, on the parents, and on examining the manner in which mutuality and trust is forged in the relationship that develops between the interdisciplinary team and parents of youngsters ages 12–21 with intellectual disability.

The research goals were: (1) To identify, describe and construct hidden and manifest aspects of collaboration between the interdisciplinary team and parents in daily practice; (2) To identify, describe, and construct behavioral expressions that comprise or are embodied in the hidden and manifest aspects of collaboration between the interdisciplinary team and parents in day-to-day practice.

4.2.1 Methodology

Qualitative research is the most suitable tool for examining and enhancing the meanings of partnership from the partners' point of view (Creswell 2002). Sandall et al. (2002) emphasize that qualitative research is particularly suited for "giving a voice to the various interested parties by listening and addressing their voice within the full context of their experiences." To understand the meaning of collaborative relations, the "interested parties" in this study are the parents and professionals who participate in the meetings. The study follows the activities of 55 interdisciplinary team members and 45 parents of special needs children. (For details on demographic characteristics of study participants, see Manor-Binyamini 2003.)

The school population was comprised of children and adolescents with intellectual disabilities, and two classes (about 20 children) of children with autism spectrum disorder. A total of 90 pupils attend this school, which serves the population residing in a very large metropolitan area in central Israel. The school day begins at 08:00 and ends at 16:00. The specific school was selected for the study because it embodied Rosenfeld's (2002) dimensions of successful learning: the objective dimension, the subjective dimension, and lack of side-effects.

4.2.1.1 Data Collection

Observations: The study demanded careful analysis of recurring aspects of all types of meetings observed, using precise methods for documenting observations, as well as verbatim transcriptions, while applying a high level of sensitivity to the unique social and interpersonal contexts in which these aspects take place. Pure ethnographic observations were conducted of formal and informal meetings of the interdisciplinary team members with the parents. The observations were open and gradually became more focused, as the components of collaboration were defined. After several months, an observation protocol was designed. All observations focused on team members and parents attending the meeting, and each meeting was fully documented. A total of 116 protocols were written, documenting a year's worth of collaboration between the interdisciplinary team and parents. Minutes taken by team members during the meetings were also collected. From a methodological perspective, the combination of research instruments served to enhance the researcher's ability to deal with issues of accessibility and to remain loyal to the point of view of both the parents and the professionals, while gathering the richest possible documentation of the social reality.

Observations included also brief (5–20 min) informal exchanges between parents and the researcher, which took place in the school playground during recess periods, and in the staffroom during school events that included the parents.

Observations of formal meetings attended by parents included the following:

(a) Hundred and eighty IEP meetings—a meeting about every student, conducted routinely at the beginning and at the end of the year. These meetings lasted between 1 and 1.5 h.

(b) Thirty meetings intended for discussing unusual events (hospitalization, return to school after hospitalization, pupil violence, non-administration of medication to a pupil, a pupil's anxiety about a certain issue).
(c) Sixteen transition meetings, i.e., meetings for the initial acquaintance between parents and the school interdisciplinary team, conducted when a child enters a special education school (7 new pupils), and farewell meetings held during an older pupil's last year in the school (9 pupils). These meetings are very emotional and a source of great stress for parents.
(d) Five meetings were conducted during the year with the Parent Representation Committee.

Interviews: To ensure a wide and diverse perspective of behavioral expressions, semi-structured interviews were conducted with 100 participants (45 parents and 55 professionals). Question structure and interview issues were identical for both groups—parents and interdisciplinary team members. Semi-structured questions enabled participants to provide the breadth and depth of information they wished to transmit. The parent group was representative of the school population in terms of pupils' ages and the grade they attended. The interviews aimed to uncover thoughts, perceptions, and opinions of professionals and parents alike about collaboration and its practical manifestation. All study participants signed an informed consent form and were notified that they could choose to terminate their participation at any time. Furthermore, anonymity and confidentiality of the data was underscored.

All interviews were recorded and transcribed. Parents were interviewed immediately after a meeting, with their prior agreement and knowledge. Their answers varied in length and depth. Professionals were interviewed throughout the year. Interviews with team members were conducted in the following order: homeroom teachers, paramedical staff, and physicians. In addition to semi-structured interviews, the study also included what Denzin (1997) termed "corridor conversations"—conversations that the researcher held with professionals, teachers, in the playground and in the staffroom during breaks or when they sat in the staffroom, and with parents visiting the school on various occasions. Most of these kinds of conversations were initiated by the professionals or the parents. Sidewalk activities (Yin 1991) provided another opportunity for informal data-gathering. These conversations were conducted with interdisciplinary team members, and sometimes with parents, when entering or leaving school, in the evenings after meetings had concluded, during school events such as holiday celebrations or at the beginning of the school year.

Document collection: A large number of documents were collected for the study. The documents can be divided into the following types: newsletter—an information bulletin sent annually to parents with information about the school structure and its operation; letters to parents—informing parents about school activities such as holidays/vacations, field-trips, special school days, and events in school (a total of 10 letters); reports on exceptional events that occurred in school—a report about serious physical or verbal violence (reports of 21 events were collected).

4.2.1.2 Data Analysis

The data analysis process included the comparison units used in qualitative analysis (Lincoln and Guba 1985), unitizing (uniting categories), categorization, data interpretation, and synthesis. In the first data analysis stage all transcriptions of verbal and nonverbal behavior were read (transcriptions of professionals and parents were read as one unit) in order to identify the minimal unit. A unit was defined as the smallest reaction of the participant that could stand on its own and that contained information which in any way related to and/or referred to the research questions (Lincoln and Guba 1985; Skrtic 1985). A reaction was defined in two ways: verbal—from a short single sentence to a long paragraph, and nonverbal behavior. A total of 35 units were identified. After units were unified, the categorization process began. Every unit was read, compared with previously read units and placed into a new or previously created category, based on its look/feel alike quality (Lincoln and Guba 1985). After deciding on the appropriate category, the unit was examined with respect to additional interview and document contexts and given a definition, thus increasing categorization accuracy. After assigning the units to the different categories, a brief rationale of their placement was noted for further examination at a later stage of the study. This was accompanied by clarification and editing of the category definitions and by justification of every unit as a specific category based on the formulated definition (Lincoln and Guba 1985). This process generated the definition of 14 categories. Possible relations between the categories were examined in the interpretation and synthesis stage of the data analysis process. Categories found to correspond to the same basis were unified into one category or theme, based on the same process described above. Themes were unified into domains and translated into aspects. Data synthesis and themes were presented as preliminary findings to an external researcher and to a research assistant, who were requested to examine coding accuracy and also to identify sub-categories from the broad categories.

4.2.1.2.1 Trustworthiness/Validity

A variety of strategies were used in the study to ensure the trustworthiness of the data collected: (a) word-by-word transcription of all research material; (b) examination of coding, conducted by an external researcher and a research assistant who designed an audit trail (Skrtic 1985) to evaluate and confirm the trustworthiness, consistency, and validity of the evidence; (c) *apparent validity*, an additional verification strategy which entailed a comprehensive examination of the data by team members and parents, to enable them to evaluate trustworthiness and validity of the interpretations and conclusions drawn from the data analysis (Lincoln, ibid; Patton 2001). The participants were asked whether their perspectives were represented and whether any important points were missing from the material presented. The respondents did not suggest any unique changes to the results obtained; (d) triangulation (Lincoln and Guba 1985) was performed for each category in the study, using various methods. Triangulation validity was tested using observations, interviews, and document collection.

4.2.2 Findings

Data analysis revealed that, in practice, collaboration took place in the organizational and the social domains (Coffey and Atkinson 1996). Organizational aspects were more manifest, while the social aspects and their behavioral expressions were more covert.

4.2.2.1 Domain 1: Organizational Aspects

The organizational domain refers to the actual meeting framework and to the inherent and constant structures that characterized the meetings: stage set, hospitality, seating arrangement, meeting structure, meeting summary, and decision-tracking.

4.2.2.1.1 The Stage Setting

The stage setting includes the physical layout, i.e., the room where the meetings took place and background items such as furniture and room decorations. According to Goffman (1959), these constitute the stage and its accessories, where—on it, in front of it, and within it—the interaction between the interdisciplinary team and parents took place. The principal's room was allocated for meetings with the participation of interdisciplinary team members and parents. The room has many windows and is furnished with armchairs and decorated with plants, creating a pleasant and warm atmosphere. The scenery in the meeting room was viewed as an important component of the success of the meetings held there.

4.2.2.1.2 Hospitality and Seating Arrangements

In interviews conducted with interdisciplinary team members and parents, they reported that a comfortable atmosphere is very important as a framework for a positive meeting. Parents were offered water or coffee when they entered the room. They were shown to their seats and sat in the center with the team members. It appears that serving coffee and refreshments eased the tension that is inevitable in the initial part of the meeting. Participants often ate and drank during the meetings. Parents perceived the offering of refreshments as a gesture of good will, because in many cultures food comprises an important component of hospitality. In the interviews, many parents indicated that they were surprised by the warm reception they received. In all teams and meetings, the chairs were arranged in a circle that also included the parents. Sitting in a circle enabled all participants to see each other and to speak face to face, creating a sense of intimacy.

4.2.2.1.3   Meeting Structure

A routine structure repeated itself in all team meetings observed—opening-discussion-closing of the meeting.

Opening of the meeting—The parents' first encounter with the entire interdisciplinary team working with their child took the form of a round of introductions. Team members introduced themselves and indicated the capacity in which they work and interact with the child. In subsequent IEP meetings or meetings about special events, the opening phase consisted of asking the parents how they felt and encouraging them to talk about their child. They were asked questions such as: how are you? How is "X?" How does s/he feel at school? In class? What does s/he tell you about school?

Many issues were presented and discussed in meetings with parents. It was apparent that the professionals knew which topics were the most important, because in all meetings the interdisciplinary team members determined the topics to be discussed and their order of importance. They presented the issues and added information from different disciplines, in order to present a clear and complete picture. Thus, for example, in IEP meetings they discussed the pupil in a holistic manner, offering information about developmental, scholastic, emotional, social, and behavioral aspects.

Closing of the meeting—In effect a meeting summary. A great deal of information was presented and discussed at these meetings. The amount of information frequently confused parents and at times they had difficulty ascertaining the degree of importance of the information communicated. Team members helped parents by briefly summarizing the issues discussed at the end of every meeting, giving the parents a sense of closure and a comprehensive picture of the child. This observation is reinforced in the words of a father who (referring to the interdisciplinary team members) noted "They know my son very well; they know precisely how to advance him—what is important and what is secondary."

4.2.2.1.4   Meeting Summary and Decision-Tracking

At all meetings, a designated team member took minutes. The minutes were typed and circulated to all team members. In many meetings, decisions were reached concerning a variety of issues and areas, for example, the referral of a pupil to a neurologist, or working with the pupil using a specific work method both at school and at home. A summary of the decisions was circulated on a monthly basis and a copy was distributed to all team members responsible for tracking decision-implementation. In most cases, the following meeting with the parents began by addressing the decisions taken at the previous meeting.

4.2.2.2 Domain 2: Social Aspects and Their Behavioral Expression

Social aspects pertain to all the personal and interpersonal aspects that contribute to effective interaction in the meeting. While these aspects are subtle, they were observed in all meetings and their behavioral expressions were delineated. A diagram displaying these aspects in detail and an example of each aspect are presented below.

4.2.2.2.1 Explaining the Professional Terminology

Interdisciplinary team members often found themselves unsure whether to use a professional term to describe the pupil, or to simplify the explanation by employing terminology that parents could understand. Team members did not avoid using professional terminology, but made a conscious effort to explain the terms. This was an informal strategy they used to ease communication with parents, based on the assumption that communication between parents and professionals might be hindered if parents did not understand the professional terms. In addition to providing an explanation, all team members frequently inquired whether parents understood the explanations provided. One of the homeroom teachers addressed this issue in the interview: "I do not think they always understand the terminology. I don't think they always understand what is going on. So we try to use language they understand. They know the meaning of the word 'functioning,' but they do not understand its significance."

It seems that by using and explaining professional terms, the team communicated respect and trust in the parent's ability to learn, thus treating parents as partners. Indeed, in many instances, parents understood the terms and used them during the meetings. It appears that parents reacted positively to this approach. During the interviews, parents emphasized that by learning the terms used by the professionals in the meetings they were able to better understand their child's condition. For example, a parent was observed saying: "I would like him to learn more functions that will help him at home and outside the home…."

Parents were found to be sensitive to professional terms. This was clearly demonstrated by a mother in an interview:

> At an early stage when we began meeting with professionals I felt that they were talking in an incomprehensible language. Do you know the amount of terms there are in this field? Think about it: ILP (individual learning program), LST (long study day), CLP (class learning program), regression…it doesn't end. It is vital that professionals explain these terms to parents, just like they do at meetings here.

Explaining professional terms enables parents to take what is said about their child and adjust it to experiences with the child at home.

4.2.2.2.2 Providing Concrete Examples

In discussing a pupil, his/her abilities, difficulties and assessment results, interdisciplinary team members generally used examples from their experiences in working with the pupil. It appears that it is easier for parents to identify and understand information that is accompanied by examples about their child. Furthermore, team members often asked parents for concrete examples, as exemplified by a homeroom teacher (in an observation): "What works with your child at home, give us an example...."

> Yesterday, after a whole year, he went to a youth movement activity entirely on his own... he crossed the street by himself.

4.2.2.2.3   Check Understanding

After providing parents with information, the team members often verified whether it was properly understood. They did so by watching the parent's face, looking for nonverbal expressions of understanding, as well as by asking direct questions as underscored by a physical therapist in an interview: "You can usually see on their faces when they have no idea what you are talking about."

This appears to be another way for team members to consolidate their relationship with parents. As professionals, they serve as mediators between professional information and parents and in that capacity they facilitate parents' ability to process the large amounts of information presented to them. Analysis of interviews with team members indicated that they viewed this strategy as a successful way to collaborate. A counselor put this very succinctly in an interview: "Many parents are wary of interfering during the meeting and therefore do not ask questions. It is very important that we, as professionals, do not assume that parents understand everything we tell them."

The greater the parents' confidence that the team listens to them, the more they express their need to understand what is being said at meetings. They do so by clarifying whether they understood what was said about their child—a major characteristic of verifying understanding. For example, a parent asked: "Is it because he doesn't get his medication in the morning that he hasn't been going to work lately...?"

4.2.2.2.4   Ask Questions

Team members asked many questions during the meetings. This activity seems like another way of helping and validating the opinions of parents as well as other team members. Questions can be classified into two types: questions requesting information or specific examples about the pupil's behaviors or learning mode, and those requesting parents' opinions. In most meetings, a gradual transition of questions posed by team members was observed, from open questions asked at the beginning of the meeting to more focused questions as the meeting progressed. The observations clearly showed that parents' comfort level in asking questions and participating in the meetings increased as the trust between team members and parents grew. It appears that all of the team members observed continued to ask the parents clarifying questions, even when they thought they understood very well what the parents had said. In a sensitive and gentle way, they communicated to parents that they were listening to what they had to say, as expected of professionals. This was evident in the words of the psychologist: "I often ask parents whether what I told them corresponds to what is happening at home and whether it accurately describes their child. They know the child so much better than I do."

Asking questions at meetings enabled parents to participate in the discussion. Furthermore, it fostered additional ideas and facilitated problem solving, by further clarifying issues and focusing problems.

Concerning this issue, a difference was observed in "transition meetings," during which parents meet for the first time with the school interdisciplinary team. It was observed that the greater the parents' feeling that they were being heard, the more questions they asked. The questions were classified into two types: those aimed at clarifying and understanding what was being said, and those posed in an attempt to solve problems and receive the team's advice. For example, a father raising his daughter alone asked: "…Up until now I helped her shower, but she's 11 years old now, and it seems to me to be inappropriate. What do you think I should do?"

4.2.2.2.5   Positive Language

Positive language has several characteristics: (a) a positive tone that is neither judgmental nor critical. Lack of blame or criticism, communicating to parents that the meeting focuses on the pupil and his or her needs; (b) the manner in which professional team members formulate their statements: on a regular basis, comments followed a structured pattern, starting with a description of the pupil's strengths that were highlighted throughout the meeting. Team members often presented ways to advance the pupils and to overcome difficulties using these strengths.

Focusing on the pupil's strengths also enabled team members to address weak points or difficulties. They did not avoid discussing loaded issues or difficulties, and moreover were very clear and direct when describing them. Team members addressed this in the interviews and underscored the importance of honesty in transmitting information to parents about their child's difficulties/disorders. Thus, for example, a therapist noted: "I do say special education because parents have the right to know and I don't want someone to say they didn't know."

The interviews, parents indicated that team members' honesty and candor was not always easy to hear, yet it consolidated their trust in the team. A mother expressed this in an interview: "…I believe them, because I know that they are not afraid of telling the truth about A's condition."

By underscoring pupils' strengths, team members succeeded in convincing parents that, despite difficulties, the pupil would succeed. Team members' ability to couple a child's strength with a weakness reflects their willingness to look for intervention methods and work strategies in their dealings with the pupils. As underscored by the principal in an interview: "Good teams always have the child's strong points in mind."

Team members also expressed their concerns to parents in a direct manner. Their tone and body language communicated this feeling: they looked at the parents while talking to them and checked to make sure their message was understood.

It is important to remember that while staff meetings are part of the team's work routine, for parents such meetings may be very emotionally charged. Therefore it is important to open the report or discussion with information emphasizing the child's strong points. Based on the observations, it appears that this strategy calmed parents, put them at ease and prevented them from becoming defensive, thus enabling them to view themselves as partners to the discussions in these meetings.

For parents, the main characteristic of positive language used by the interdisciplinary team had to do with emphasis on the school's investment in their children. For example, in an interview with a mother she noted:

> …The first time I participated in a team meeting I was surprised: eleven team members sat there, can you imagine—eleven team members all sitting and talking and discussing my son for a whole hour. It gives you the feeling that they care, that they take their job seriously.

Another mother stated: "They consider every request I make."

4.2.2.2.6 Professional Expertise

Professional expertise, as perceived by the team members, is reflected in their serious attitude towards meetings. This seriousness, as they see it, is demonstrated by the fact that they prepare for the meetings in advance. In other words, all team members are familiar with the pupil, have conducted an assessment, are aware of the pupil's strengths and weaknesses, and have defined specific goals in working with the pupil. In the words of the psychiatrist:

> Everyone does his or her job and then when we meet to discuss the child, then every team member has extensive information in their area of expertise, but team members are open to the opinions of others…I think that the bottom line here at school is that the team and the teachers respect each other's judgment… and we want to do what is best for the children.

Team members demonstrated professional expertise through their acquaintance with the pupils and their needs, freeing them to listen to the discussion rather than being preoccupied by the need to look up information on the pupil's status and progress. When professionals are familiar with a pupil, they do not have to glance at the documents or remember what they wanted to say. Thus, they are free to focus their attention on the parents and on other team members, to look at them and ensure that they understand what is being said. Expertise enables the meetings to flow smoothly, facilitates informed decisions, and paves the ways for a clear focus, a useful summary of the information presented, and an effective discussion. As the psychologist explained: "If you are an expert and sure of yourself, then it frees you to be a better listener…you simply listen better and this enables you to be more open to the analysis."

According to the parents, team members' expertise was reflected in knowing and understanding the class study program, the pupil's individual study program, as well as the team's work with their child. In certain instances, parents were observed coming to meetings prepared with points they would like to address, and also taking notes during the meeting.

4.2.2.2.7 Focus

Meetings of the interdisciplinary team with parents are attended by many experts, and numerous issues are raised and discussed. Therefore, it was quite surprising to note that all of the meetings observed over the entire year ended on time. The meetings opened with a warm and cordial introduction, immediately after which team members conducted the meeting. It was evident that team members were well aware of the importance of the time element for the parents, as reflected in the words of a mother in the interview: "I am grateful to the team for making an effort to end the meeting at the designated time; it feels good to know that they value my time."

Complying with the timetable was possible because team members were focused. Each member in turn presented information to parents in a clear and organized manner. In the interviews, all professionals noted the importance of adhering to the meeting's objectives and focus. In the interviews, parents also noted that focusing on the issue at hand enabled them to follow the discussion and understand what was said by the team members.

Another expression of focus was the informative summary made by team members for the benefit of the parents. In each meeting, one team member assumed this informal role; in the study, this individual was known as the "integrator." This team member, who was not formally appointed to this position, summarized and integrated all information presented during the meeting. The summary enabled team members and parents to organize everything that was discussed and presented into a comprehensive picture, to focus the discussion and decide on goals for working with the pupil as well as on other issues. This feature was very important because parents obtained a great deal of information at these meetings. The following is an example of a summary given by a psychologist:

> …several issues were raised here: I think we all agree that R has good functioning ability, and we saw this in the occupational diagnoses, but this does not manifest itself because he does not come to school. Three weeks have passed since the beginning of the year and he still he stays home from school every day. The most important goal in working with him now is to encourage him to come to work….

Parents noted two characteristics that demonstrated the well-defined focus of the meetings: the fact that at each meeting clear goals were set for working with their child, and the fact that the professionals were indeed listening to the parents and setting these goals in line with their description of the child's needs. Most parents addressed this issue in the interview. One mother noted: "Ever since my daughter has been in this school she is continuously progressing in academic, social, or occupational areas. They constantly set goals and everybody works towards achieving the same goal."

Concerning goals adjusted to the child's needs, a father said:

> ...The truth is that I was scared a few months ago when they discussed my son's army recruitment; I was sure he would not be up to it. Now, I see how he waits for Wednesday in order to go fulfill his army duty and how happy he is when he gets back. When I heard his commander speak on "Employer Day" I understood that they know my son very well, that his placement suits him and is right for him.

4.2.2.2.8   Balance in the Interdisciplinary Power Structure

Balance in the interdisciplinary power structure takes place at the informal and covert level of communication and is observed mainly during decision-making processes. During the decision-making process or while discussing a pupil, team members tended to support each other. No single team member ever dominated the discussion or tried to force their point of view on others. In the interviews held with the team members, they described a sense of balance among them. In cases of disagreement, they focused on the discussion rather than on power struggles. A speech therapist noted in the interview that discussions are characterized by a genuine desire to learn more rather than to prove who is right. The observations revealed that team members did not take disagreement between team members or between team members and parents personally and therefore did not feel angry or hurt by team members or parents. Team members viewed differences of opinion as learning opportunities and challenges.

4.2.2.2.9   Clear Definition of Parents' Role

The way in which team members perceived the parents played a vital role in team meetings. Teams expected parents to participate in meetings and viewed their attendance as part of their parental responsibilities. In other words, they felt that part of their role as professionals was to provide support and encouragement to parents and, by doing so, to help them become involved partners in the processes taking place at the meetings. Team members interpreted parents' lack of participation as a failure on their part to fulfill their role as professionals. A speech therapist said in an interview: "We work very hard to bring parents to the point that they ask questions. We always want parents to be more involved."

Team members perceived parents as experts on their child, with important information about him/her. This information relates to the pupil's development, education, and recreational activities and was considered a significant contribution to the meeting. It appears that treating parents as experts on the subject of their child and attaching importance to the information they presented led parents to actively participate in meetings. Professionals achieved this through both verbal and nonverbal behavior, as observed by the researcher at a meeting:

> Rather than looking down at the parent or sending their pronouncements to float randomly through the airwaves, the team members gave the mother their full attention. They leaned

forward in their seats naturally, looked at her directly, and made eye contact. Their gestures seemed calming, and without words they showed her that she was important and that her presence was important.

The parents saw themselves as responsible for their children. They conveyed this by giving voice to the child's feelings, desires, problems, anxieties, and frustrations, experienced both at home and at school. In an observation of a meeting, a mother was documented saying: "...She doesn't like gym class; she says the other children badger her."

4.2.2.2.10   Making Room for Parents' Feelings

The team members observed in the study made room for, validated, and focused on parents' feelings. With parents who experienced anxiety about their child's entering a special education school, the team tended to focus on the parents' feelings and in doing so enabled the discussion to continue, as demonstrated by the counselor asking a parent directly: "You seem anxious about the word *retardation*, is there any question you might have that we can answer?"

Team members spoke softly, yet professionally. They looked directly at the parents and listened carefully to their answers. In doing so, they communicated that parents' feelings were important and relevant, and frequently addressed those feelings and the parents' questions. Parents' comments and suggestions were weighed seriously and team members often asked additional questions or requested more details, verbally amplifying every comment and insight received from the parents. In addressing this aspect in the interviews, parents noted that they felt their opinions were valued. As the meeting continued, it was common to observe increased parent participation. When parents felt that their opinions were important, their active participation in meetings increased and their trust in the professional team was enhanced. This in turn laid the foundation for implementing team recommendations or supporting and continuing work with the child at home. Conversely, by exhibiting defensive behavior or ignoring parents' comments, team members communicated disregard for parents' feelings, causing them to become distanced and to withdraw their participation and contribution to the meeting.

According to parents, this component is characterized by a feeling that it is legitimate to express anger, fear, and sadness. In the words of an interviewed mother: "This team does not become alarmed by anything said in the room. Over the years, I have been angry at them, sometimes I cried, but they don't get scared...."

4.2.2.2.11   Respect

Respect is an important element in meetings, as it contributes to the development of positive relations. It appears that respect is built on the basis of joint work and a prolonged acquaintance. These feelings were voiced by team members in the interviews and were also evident in the observations. Mutual respect among team members was reflected in their behavior during meetings. They listened genuinely to each other and often asked questions or for each other's opinion. They also demonstrated respect towards parents. Observations of body language and behavior at meetings created a continuing and compelling sense of respectful behavior among all the participants. Team members consistently exhibited politeness. They spoke calmly, describing problem behaviors in a way that expressed concern. At no time during the observations were team members observed expressing anger or blame. When communicating information to parents, their genuineness and concern were evident and conspicuous. The teams created an atmosphere characterized by warmth and support, concomitant with a high level of professionalism. Respect towards parents did not hinder team members from discussing children's problems or difficulties. To the contrary, they presented difficulties clearly and unequivocally because, as they claimed, parents have a right to receive information about their child, even if the information may not be positive. At the same time, they were nonjudgmental when doing so. In the interviews, parents reported a sense of relief that they were able to discuss any issue with the team members, including their own concerns which they had concealed for a long time. It appears to be easier for parents to accept and digest information when it is presented professionally and in a caring manner. Furthermore, they feel that they are being treated respectfully.

In both observations and interviews, parents continuously used the word *respect*. It was specifically used in two contexts: respect accorded to pupils, and parents' feeling that they were respected by team members. Observations and interviews indicated that parents felt respected when the team was attentive to their ideas and showed a willingness to implement their suggestions. Parents perceived the team's interest and caring towards pupils as reflecting respect towards their child. One father noted in an interview: "When A was hospitalized for 1 week, it was touching to see the teacher and personal assistant visit him every day. After all, it's not part of their job" (Fig. 4.3).

4.2.3   Conclusions

The study presented here attempted to examine components of collaboration between professionals and parents and to delineate aspects constituting the foundation for effective collaboration as it takes place in practice, on a daily basis, in the special education context. Understanding and awareness of behaviors embodied in collaboration are important due to the inherent differences between the partners: parents represent the primary, emotional, and subjective system, while interdisciplinary school team members represent the secondary, functional, and objective system. The difference between the two systems is fundamental and suggests an inbuilt conflict, which could create tension and hinder collaboration. This inherent difficulty is often reflected in emotionally laden situations experienced by parents. In the meetings and in the interviews, parents displayed a variety of feelings ranging from anger and fear to sadness and confusion. These feelings were overt and their

Behavioral Expressions

Social Aspects

Organizational Aspects

Collaboration

Professionals: Listen genuinely to what is said in meeting, consult during meeting, demonstrate politeness, speak calmly, create warm personal atmosphere

Parents: Try to understand professional terms and how they relate to their child

Professionals: Use professional terms, explain them and give examples

Parents: Express their appreciation towards the team for respecting them and their children

Professionals expected to respect, validate and support parent's feelings, tone of voice soft but professional, treat what parents say seriously, verbal empowerment of parent's statements

Parents: Express a range of feelings

Parents: Present and describe their child using concrete examples

Professionals: Provide information about pupil's strengths, weaknesses and evaluation results along with examples from team members work with the pupil

Explain professional terminology

Respect

Provide concrete examples

Parents: Try to understand what is being said as it relates to their child

Professionals: Team Members expected and urged to encourage, assist and support parent participation in the meeting, view parents as experts on their child

Make room for parent's feelings

Stage set

Check understanding

Professionals: Observe parents' facial expressions, verbally assess parents' understanding, ask direct questions

Parents: Represent the child and give voice to his/her needs and concerns

Clear definition of parent's role

Ask questions

Parents: Transition' meetings differ from other types of meetings; ask clarifying questions and questions aimed at solving problems and receiving advice

Professionals: Support, no professional dominates the discussion, team members do not try to prove that they are right, differences of opinion among professionals seen as learning opportunities

Balance in the Interdisciplinary power structure

Hospitality and seating arrangement

Summary and decision making

Positive language

Professionals: Ask questions aimed at obtaining details or specific examples of behavior or learning mode. Ask questions to hear their opinion. Gradual shift from open to focused questions

Parents:

Focus

Professional expertise

Parents: Underscore the school's investment in their child

Professionals: Time management of meeting, comply with timetable, focus on meeting goals, informative summary of what was said to provide a comprehensive picture

Parents: Set clear goals suited to their child's needs

Professionals: Team members prepare in advance and come prepared to meetings. They are familiar with the pupil, prepared a diagnosis and planned work goals

Parents: Familiar with and understand the class study program and the 'IEP-Individual Education Plan'

Professionals: 'Non -judgmental' tone, lack of blame; underscore pupil's strengths, report on difficulties and loaded issues. Clear and honest description of pupil's difficulties

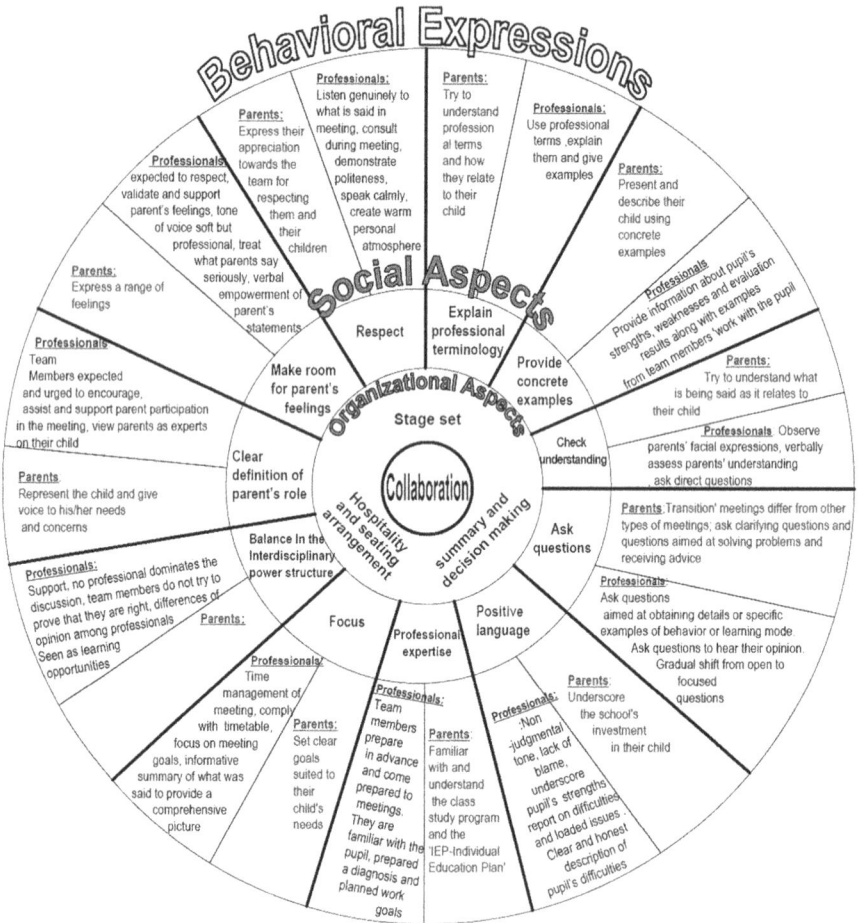

Fig. 4.3 A schematic summary of practical collaboration between experts and parents in an existing special education school. Adapted from Manor-Binyamini (2004)

intensity was often strong and dramatic. The study showed that despite the fundamental differences between the two systems, building collaboration between parents and professionals is possible. Collaboration is comprised of multidimensional organizational and social aspects and a range of behaviors occurring simultaneously in the two-way interaction between parents and the interdisciplinary team. *It appears that professionals must have the ability to demonstrate all social behaviors simultaneously in their meetings with parents.* The study reinforces the conclusions reached by Stoner et al. (2005) concerning the complexity of collaboration with parents. Identifying and evaluating skills and behaviors of professionals that can facilitate such collaboration continues to be of vital importance. (The study has several limitations as well as implications at the policy, research, and application levels. For a description, see Manor-Binyamini 2004.)

To sum up this subchapter, I believe we can define *collaboration*, much like Freire (1970) defined dialogue, as "a genuine act of creation." The current study demonstrates that such a creation is possible, and attempts to lay the foundation for its implementation and development in the context of the interactions between professionals and parents.

4.3 Collaboration Between Professionals and Parents in Indigenous Communities

The definitions, the features, and the practices outlined in the previous sections of this chapter are all informed by Western culture. Hence, when applying them towards collaboration between parents and professionals in indigenous communities, some of these concepts may be useful while others might not, given the diversity of cultures and factors related to the context that characterizes each indigenous community. These factors and community-sensitive issues inevitably affect both parties: the parents as well as the professionals who work in the special education schools in indigenous communities. These factors and their effect on the parties involved could influence the nature of their collaboration within the schools, and therefore they should be identified and addressed. This section concentrates first on presenting and explaining the issues and factors which should be taken into account, and then examines the potential outcomes for all the participants: children, parents, and professionals.

4.3.1 Issues and Factors That Affect Collaboration Between Parents from Indigenous Communities and the Professionals Who Care for Children with Disabilities at School

Many issues and factors may affect the motivation, the ability, and the willingness of parents of children with disabilities to enter into a relationship of collaboration with professionals working in the schools. This section attempts to answer the question: could the characteristics unique to indigenous communities affect the collaboration between parents and professionals working in special education schools, and if so, what might be the nature that effect?

Previous chapters have reviewed the existential challenges with which indigenous populations all over world must contend (see Chaps. 1 and 2). These challenges include health risks, high illiteracy rates, geographical constraints (rural or remote locations), poverty, political marginalization, and dispossession, all factors which play a part in the lack of available means of transportation and the need for more extensive support services. In addition, we have seen (in Chap. 2) that each indigenous community is guided by its particular indigenous knowledge (i.e., concepts and behavioral norms that have been passed from one generation to the next) and its own indigenous psychology (principal beliefs and guidelines for explaining how the world works and the place of human life within this system). It is inevitable that these issues shape the ways in which parents construct and view education and schools.

4.3.1.1 Existential Challenges Faced by Indigenous Populations and Their Potential Effects on Collaboration with School Professionals

This section takes an in-depth look at the existential challenges faced by indigenous communities throughout the world and considers their influence on the day-to-day living conditions of the parents, which in turn affect their interactions with school professionals. Equally, lack of awareness of these challenges on the part of the school professionals will undoubtedly affect their attitudes, actions, and reactions as they seek to interact and collaborate with these parents.

Political subjugation, legal and social discrimination, isolation, and exclusion, loss of language and loss of lands—this "historical heritage," bequeathed to indigenous communities by past government policies have left indigenous people disempowered. Indigenous peoples' lack of political status is inherently linked to poor socioeconomic conditions, which correlates with increased health risks. These in turn are exacerbated by indigenous communities' remote geographical locations, which result in difficulty accessing health and education facilities. Poor health and education go hand-in-hand with high rates of illiteracy, and lack of education perpetuates the poverty cycle.

These conditions have a strong influence on the day-to-day lives of the parents of children with disabilities. Collaborating with professionals at the school means that the parents first have to get to the school, which in itself can present multiple challenges, whether of giving up on a chance to earn their daily bread, leaving infants at home, or finding transportation—and money for transportation—to the school. In addition, professionals who provide services in the form of education and healthcare are part of the state or local government and, as such, bear the legacy of previous governments' acts of disempowerment. In other words, many indigenous people have learned over generations to be distrustful and fearful of government services.

Without understanding the challenges these parents face, daily and existentially, we cannot understand what it means to ask for parents' collaboration (Begay et al. 1999). To date, relatively little attention has been paid to the impact that these core conditions have on the attempts of special education schools to work with indigenous communities. In contrast, there is increasing interest in the subject of *culture* in the special education professional literature.

4.3.1.2 Indigenous and Western Culture and Psychology: The Effects on the Potential Collaboration Between Parents in Indigenous Communities and School Professionals

Cultural knowledge is unconsciously acquired and passed from generation to generation. Thus, the concepts that underlie a community's preferences and behaviors may differ dramatically from one cultural to another.

4.3.1.2.1   Interpersonal Communication

Examples of culturally bound behaviors include the customary methods of greeting (formal versus informal); the type of dress (professional versus informal); degree of eye contact when interacting (direct contact versus looking down or away); the person to whom inquiries are directed (mother, father' elder' other family member); and method through which information is gathered (orally versus written, structured versus open-ended questions). Differences in communication, especially in nonverbal communication (behavior), means that a gesture can be interpreted very differently by different cultures, which, of course, can have an adverse effect on efforts to forge a meaningful relationship between individuals of different cultures. For example, a parent's silence can be attributed as much to the professional's imposition of the parameters for discourse as to differences in interpersonal communication styles. Native American and Asian parents, who place great value on personal stoicism and containment of emotion, may prefer to remain silent rather than discuss with unknown professionals what they consider to be family problems (Lau 2010), while in the case of African American parents, silence can convey a lack of trust in authority figures (Harry et al. 2005).

4.3.1.2.2   Special Education and the Service Professional

The mandate for parents' collaboration and participation in discussions with professionals at school directly contradicts the traditional notion of professional as expert. The idea that parents are also experts about their child can be problematic for professionals who have been trained to believe that their knowledge gives them authority to make decisions about a student's education. The internal conflict is even more bewildering from the perspective of the indigenous parents, as many non-Western cultures tend to view the professional as the source of unquestionable knowledge, and therefore expect the professional to deliver an expert opinion in a categorical manner (Cho et al. 2003; Lai and Ishiyama 2004). They certainly do not expect to be collaborators in the decision-making process. By contrast, professional staff members who do expect to have the parents' collaboration, often take for granted certain beliefs that pertain to Western culture, and to their professional culture in particular: (a) Parents have the right to know and are entitled to access to the same knowledge that the professionals have about their child; (b) parents will advocate for their child by exercising these rights; (c) all parents are equally knowledgeable and have a "shared understanding" (Harry 1992). Parents from indigenous communities often do not have this shared understanding about the school and may not have the means to learn. Nor are they likely to serve as advocates for their children; in fact, as mentioned, they tend to defer to the professional.

The professionals working in special education schools bring yet another inherent cultural bias to the collaboration: the cultural underpinnings of special education schools. Bullivant (1993) explained the powerful relationship between the larger macro culture, i.e., the establishment's education system, and the special education schools that function as a subsystem within the social establishment. First, he identified these institutions as a "major interrelated systems of social roles and norms (rules) organized to satisfy important social and human needs" (p. 31). Accordingly, one of the roles of the schools that form this subsystem is to reflect the "beliefs, values, and ideas" of the greater education system, serving as a means to an end dictated by the national-level, macro establishment.

The process through which professionals prepare to become staff members in the special education schools draws most heavily on the macro society's cultural belief systems, as it provides the framework on which the field of education is founded. Induction into special education, then, is accomplished by building on the implicit knowledge base of the macroculture, through formal instruction in the theoretical and applied knowledge of the field and, finally, through practical experience in schools (Skrtic 1991). In most situations, the cultural rules of the establishment are not explicitly taught to the inductees, precisely because the insiders themselves may not be aware that they are functioning according to the built-in rules of the system. As in the transmission of any cultural heritage, the process of induction is a covert one. Bowers (1995) referred to this knowledge as the "taken-for-granted" beliefs that are experienced as "the natural order of things." Special education is full of such embedded beliefs. Indeed, already in their education and training, professionals will have learned to operate using particular models (see Chap. 3—on the role of experts). Every one of those models was studied and researched in Western cultures, and their applicability for working with parents from indigenous communities has not been studied.

Hence, in special education schools, the result of such beliefs is that parents who do not share or value the cultural framework (as in the case of parents from indigenous communities) on which special education policies and practices are built are all too often alienated and excluded from collaboration in the treatment of their children's difficulties (for a comprehensive review on this subject, see Harry 2008). When parents are excluded, children's development is stunted, and attempts to proffer remediation and support result in minimal progress for children and frustration for professionals and parents alike (Kalyanpur and Harry 2012, p. 3).

4.3.1.2.3 The Conceptions of Disability and its Causes

The concept of disability is perceived of as a Western concept, and has no parallels in the perspectives of most indigenous communities around the world: Harry (1992) stated that disabilities are culturally defined. Every culture has different parameters for typical and atypical development. Some cultures accept a wider range of diversity in behavior and development. For example, if a child has a communication problem and that condition does not prevent the child from helping with the family household chores, the parents may not think of the child as "disabled."

Many tribes believe that speaking about a disability gives it power to manifest itself in human form. For example, if an individual is mentally healthy, she is considered to be also physically healthy, even though the same individual may have an impairment that has an effect on a particular physical function. Native Americans often define the term *disability* in terms of a relationship between individuals with unequal abilities and not as a consequence of medical or environmental conditions (Pichette et al. 1999).

Regardless of either the manifestations (cognitive or physical) or the genetic etiologies of disability, it constitutes a sociocultural phenomenon. The manner in which it is defined and labeled, the adaptability and responses of parents, perceived difficulties and opportunities, as well as the values attributed to differences in abilities—these are all linked to other societal characteristics. Likewise, the professional practices and institutions that develop to address disability are all social and cultural constructions that have evolved over time, at multiple levels and within particular historical and political contexts (Stiker 1999; Albrecht et al. 2001).

One of the typical differences between Western and non-Western conceptions of disability is the importance of the community and the effect of the disability on the individual's ability to carry out the functions central to the particular community. Edgerton (1970) found that among the Manus of New Guinea, for example, the loss of an arm was much more of a disability and much more stigmatizing than the inability to read, because being able to handle a canoe was a necessary survival skill. Ethnographic explorations of disability suggest that a child may be considered disabled if she must depend on others for assistance to fulfill their culturally expected roles. For example, in the Bedouin community, an individual whose ability to walk was impaired would be at a disadvantage in this nomadic culture.

Another major conceptual difference between indigenous and non-indigenous cultures is the way they explain the cause of disability. Within aboriginal or Native American cultures, for example, life is viewed as a series of concentric circles, like ripples on a lake. Circles of life energy are believed to exist within people, surround them, and make up relationships. Harmony and balance in all relationships, between all the circles, is necessary for the survival of all life. This belief system was further described in an exploration of disability within the Dine (Navajo) culture in the Southwestern USA by Frankland et al. (2004). Mind-body-spirit harmony is considered central to personal and family well-being. Disability is attributed to disharmony with the universe. In some cultures, disability is understood to be a spiritual phenomenon, a manifestation of the "evil eye." Curses and other metaphors of spiritual malevolence also are seen as common causes for sickness and disability among many African, Hmong, Jewish Oriental, Native American, and Latin American parents (Kalyanpur and Harry 2012).

Beliefs about the causes of disability can also affect a parent's perspective on whether a condition is chronic. Among many non-Western cultures, time is cyclical and therefore, infinite. Danseco noted that among parents who believe in reincarnation, disability is perceived as a temporary condition when viewed along several possible lives (1997, p. 44).

Different cultures attach very different meanings to the presence of disabilities or at-risk conditions. Views related to disability and its causation range from those which emphasize the role of fate to those which place responsibility on the person or the individual's family (Hanson et al. 1990). In some cultures, parents might be blamed for the child's disability. Some may see the disability as a punishment for sins; others may view it a result of some action the mother or father took while the mother was pregnant. Still other groups may attribute causation to mind-body imbalances or the presence of evil spirits in the child's body (Hanson et al. 1990).

In light of the fact that the concept of disability is defined differently across cultures (Fadiman 1997; Lo 2005), when the cultural framework of service providers differs from that of the parents they serve, the potential for cross-cultural miscommunication is extremely high. It is therefore important for professionals to consider how parents perceive disability and the cause of disability: equipping service professionals with this knowledge can have a great impact on the motivation of members of indigenous communities to seek support services and the types of interventions they are likely seek (Danseco 1997).

4.3.1.2.4 Differences Between Indigenous and Western Culture and Psychology

When parents of indigenous communities and professionals working in special education schools that represent the Western culture attempt to join forces, they each rely on a different cultural system, a difference that could lead to conflicts between the participants. For example, an Aboriginal worldview sees people as integral to the world with humans having a seamless relationship with nature, which includes seas, land, rivers, mountains, flora, and fauna (Te Ahukaramu 2002). As mentioned, in the Native American worldview, harmony with the universe is considered essential to humans' well-being.

Thus, the goals of parenting in any culture are geared to prepare children to live within the framework defined by the parents' worldview. Similarly, the role of the parent, the psychological patterns of parents' reactions to stress, and their coping mechanisms also must cohere with their worldview. Every one of these aspects has an effect on the parents' childrearing practices, on their willingness to collaborate, and on the quality and effectiveness of the interactions with support-service professionals.

4.3.1.2.5 Parenting, Child Rearing Practices and Child Development

Parents of children with disabilities in indigenous communities have a concept of parenting which is different from the way parenting is perceived in Western society and which is reflected in the way they raise their children. The study of Westerman and Wettinfer (1997) provides a pertinent example of differences between Aboriginal and White Australian child rearing practices. Table 4.5 represents a summary of information from various texts about Aboriginal women's roles in their community and their child rearing practices.

Such differences should be noted, as they might lead to conflict between professionals and parents, due to the fact that special education practices are based on the assumption that children's developmental milestones are biologically determined. These milestones then serve as a yardstick which ensures that the measurement of development is scientifically objective and therefore universal applicable. Thus,

Table 4.5 Overview of differences between Aboriginal and White Australian child rearing practices

Areas of development	Aboriginal Australian children	White Australian children
Childcare responsibilities	Shared usually by the large, extended family group Babies are treated with extreme indulgence by everyone in the family. In the extended family there are often others to relieve the pressure on the mother Young children are seen as having the capacity to demand, e.g., "She will cry if she is hungry"	This role is usually taken by the child's mother with input from the father. In the nuclear family, the mother is often has to cope on her own Babies are encouraged to adopt a regular routine which is endorsed by the main caregiver Young children are seen as helpless and all decisions are made for them, "Mum knows best"
Oral development	Little oral obedience-training	Oral obedience-training begins early, e.g., understanding words such as "no," "stop" and "naughty"
The first steps to independence	Physical interaction—children in family group Sleeping—in any room or place Young children are allowed to move away from adults. Usually in the care of older children Older siblings and other children mix together out of mother's sight Children accept responsibility for each other with no adults present	Physical interaction—when the child is awake Sleeping—often put to sleep in a room away from the family or lying in a basinet or bouncer Young children are expected to stay close to adults. Children are assumed "lost" if they are out of the mother's sight Siblings and other young children mix together but everyone knows that Mum is in charge
Physical skills	Can develop without restraints of adults. There are few verbal commands by adults; even if are present. Children learn capacity to perform feats to hurt themselves.	Children are less skilled physically Adults are expected to warn and to set limits, e.g., "be careful"; "that's high enough." Adults use lots of verbal commands Children are not expected to cope with hurt or fear by themselves; adults have the expectation that they know best
Play/activities involvement	These are of the child's choosing and continue to be used until the child wishes to stop	These are often chosen or suggested by the parent or caregiver. There is encouragement to do particular jobs, e.g., putting toys away and washing hands
	Competition is not encouraged. The guiding principle is to pursue whatever is best for the family/group	Competition is often encouraged by caregivers, between siblings and peers. There is an idea of "doing what is best of the individual"

Adapted from Westerman and Wettinfer (1997, pp. 9–10)

most Western adaptive behavior scales are developed on the understanding that children acquire mastery over specific tasks at particular ages (Scherzer 2009). However, cross-cultural research points to the cultural specificity of developmental expectations or timetables. A comparison of mothers' timetables across cultural communities revealed variations in the acquisition of skills which are supposedly "biologically predetermined," such as infant crawling and toilet training, as well as in the learning of the more socially defined skills, such as verbal communication (Burchinal et al. 2010; Scherzer 2009).

The implications of the variations outlined here is that the expectations of professionals working in schools that are founded on Western regarding proper rearing practices are necessarily different from those of parents from indigenous communities. Judgments about good parenting skills or rearing practices, as defined by the school culture, may alienate parents of indigenous communities and diverse cultural heritages. Parents whose rearing practices differ from those of the school culture may not trust school personnel, and they may experience confusion (Manning and Lee 2001) and resentment (De Carvalho 2001).

Professionals who remain uninformed about such cultural differences are likely to encounter difficulties when working with parents from indigenous communities. The traditional Western paradigm of professionalism includes the implicit assumption that professionals have the expert knowledge to evaluate, classify, and provide appropriate special education services to students who have disabilities. Such technical rationalism also assumes that this expertise can be used systematically to accumulate objective knowledge about reality (Skrtic 1995). The concept of objectivity is essentially Western, as Pedersen (1981) noted "Western culture emphasizes objectivity and the scientific method of discovering the truth as more valid and reliable that subjective and spiritual access to knowledge" (1981, p. 324). This "truth knowledge" rejects the possibility of alternative points of view, such as the parents' everyday (indigenous) knowledge about their child's difficulties. If traditionally experts have tended to dismiss parents' knowledge as subjective and anecdotal (Turnbull et al. 2007), the professional who is not educated regarding the alternative views contributed by indigenous parents may easily relapse into that "traditional model," which in turn could jeopardize the relationship with the parents and the intervention intended for the child's benefit.

4.3.1.2.6 Setting Goals for the Intervention Program

Just as parenting goals of parents from indigenous communities reflect their psychology and worldview, the goals set for the intervention will also be affected by their particular cultural psychology. Setting goals for individuals does not occur in a social or cultural vacuum (Harry 2008). Thus, the differences between the indigenous and the Western worldviews are thus most likely to emerge during a discussion regarding the goals one is trying to achieve when working with the student.

The cornerstone for goal setting in special education is the formulation of the Individual Education Program, that is, the intervention program required by law to eligible students from ages 3 to 21 years. The IEP is the heart of the intervention process, and it must be prepared and presented as a written document delineating the special education and related services to be provided. An IEP must include the student's present level of performance and disability classification, the recommended program placement, related services to be provided, a timeline for the projected goals to be accomplished, annual goals and short-term instructional objectives, and evaluation methods (Mernis and Leininger 1992). The *IEP meeting* is the formal conference during which an IEP is developed from both parental and professional input, and thus it is also the primary forum for collaboration between parents and professionals.

However, the very framework on which the IEP is based highlights the different worldviews of the collaborating parties: in the indigenous community, the group is the most important unit, and as mentioned, goals are set to accommodate the needs of the group, whereas the IEP places the individual in the center, and the goals are defined according to the needs of the individual. Indeed, the very approach of the special education school presupposes the importance of outcomes such as individual diagnosis/assessment, planning, individual education programs, and other adapted individualized intervention techniques.

The Western emphasis on individualism assumes that children with disabilities have rights and that they have the right to maximize their potential. These values are tied to the ideals of upward social mobility and freedom of choice. Educational programming for children with disabilities incorporates these assumptions by planning towards a normal routine of life, which would include the same activities and developmental life-cycle experiences as those available to people without disabilities. An interrelated goal is to provide children opportunities and guide them to make their own choices on these issues.

Clearly, these two different—if not opposing—worldviews affect the working process, the working plans, and their results. Professional interactions that lack awareness of these cultural underpinnings have the potential to arouse conflicts, especially since, as shown previously, parents may stress their satisfaction with the current state of their child, whether because the child is functional in terms of community participation, or due to shame or a need to keep family matters private. These kinds of conflict might lead to a lower rate of parent participation in IEP meetings, which in turn might lead to a scenario where the work that is being done at the schools doesn't meet the real needs of the student and thus might even stunt the child's development.

Still other factors underscore the cultural sensitivity required if these IEP meetings are to proceed successfully. For example, even parents from indigenous communities who are interested in participating in the planning and development of their children's IEP might feel uncomfortable and out of place, because of the differences in their social, cultural, and linguistic characteristics, and because of the differences that stem from the living conditions that characterize their daily lives. This discomfort can be aroused, for example, by the fact that legally, school professionals are obligated to provide parents with written information describing the IEP. However, one of the cultural assumptions embedded in this legal directive is the assumption of literacy. As mentioned in Chap. 1, many people in indigenous communities are not literate. Placing the parents in this untenable position, which clearly fails to recognize their hardships, on the one hand, and their vulnerability in the unfamiliar culture of the special education school, on the other, certainly has the potential to undermine the efforts of collaboration.

4.3.1.2.7 Time

Another example of the effect of the differences between indigenous and Western psychology is related to the understanding of time. Although Western law requires that the process of setting up the IEP be completed within 30–60 days, this time constraint may not be in the best interests of the child and parents. Establishing rapport (e.g., having conversations, interpreting, sharing, accepting) with parents and taking the time to introduce them to the special education system and process is a recommended strategy on which school professionals rely (Chan 1990; Kalyanpur and Rao 1991; Lynch and Hanson 1998). The initial contact with the parents is a critical period of time for professionals to get to know the child and parent/family. In this critical period of time, professionals can explain the terminology, explain the diagnosis and the intricacy of special education and related services, share their expectations, and understand the family's expectations, hopes, and aspirations.

Another aspect of time is that professionals may see themselves as short-term providers, who spend a limited period of time with children. Parents see the care of their child as an ongoing and lifelong commitment. These different expectations need to be addressed and bridged.

4.3.2 The Impact on Collaboration

4.3.2.1 Impact on the Parents

4.3.2.1.1 School Culture Shock

Culture shock occurs when a person, profession parent, family, or group from one culture is attempting to function within an unfamiliar culture. Disorientation occurs from not understanding the language, customs, beliefs, and expectations of the other culture. School culture shock is the result of a series of disorienting encounters that occur when an individual's basic values, beliefs, and patterns of behavior are challenged by a different set of values, beliefs, and patterns of behavior. Culture shock occurs when the strategies that the individual uses to solve problems, make decisions, and interact positively are not effective and when the individual feels an overwhelming sense of discomfort in the environment (Drain and Hall 1986). As a result of different behaviors, different values, and different interpretations of those behaviors, due to culture, ethnicity, language, or locality, contextual tensions may emerge in the interactions between parents and professionals. Confusion and tension lead to discomfort, which could cause both parties to withdraw. The discomfort may manifest itself in emotional or physical ways, such as lack of cooperation, communication, resistance, frustration, anger, depression, lethargy, aggression, or illness. In any of these states, it is difficult for the individual to take constructive action. Parents from indigenous communities experience culture shock as they attempt to negotiate a new culture, For many parents from indigenous communities who have children with disabilities, entering the culture of special education school is like landing in a foreign country, where they experience cultural chook. The same can be said of some of the professionals.

4.3.2.2   Impact on the School Professionals

4.3.2.2.1   Cultural Blindness

A lack of awareness and understanding of the indigenous community's existential challenges, historical heritage, living conditions, and indigenous knowledge and psychology, with emphasis on the concepts of child rearing, parenting, and disability, the professional is culturally blind. By definition, cultural blindness serves as grounds for conflict and undoubtedly inhibits collaboration.

4.3.2.3   The Impact on the Collaborating Parties

4.3.2.3.1   Conflict

As we can see from above, factors affecting the parents' collaboration are complex and intertwined, and can lead to a conflict on many fundamental issues that inform the collaboration (e.g., view of disability, knowledge about disability, accessibility of support services).

Parents who are unfamiliar or inexperienced in the ways of the support-service systems that they encounter need to make adjustments, as do the profession who are unfamiliar and inexperienced in the ways of the parents they meet (Lynch and Hanson 1998, p. 36). As a result, while working with the parents, professionals may experience some of the same emotional turmoil that the parents feel towards the new culture; anger, frustration, and a desire to pull away are typical reactions.

Recent research indicates that one potential source of conflict revolves around the cultural beliefs held by educators. At times, these beliefs are in opposition to beliefs held by the parents who come from differing cultural backgrounds (Garcia et al. 2000). Culture, language, ethnicity, and race are not the only determinants of one's values, beliefs, and behaviors. Every one of the issues and factors that have been presented herein all exert a powerful influence over how individuals view themselves and how parents and professionals function.

4.3.2.4   The Impact on the Children

Child Development—Every one of the factors considered in this chapter might hinder or even prevent collaboration between professionals and parents in special education schools. Inability to collaborate has a direct effect on assessment, planning, and implementing work plans for the child. A process that is derailed due to lack of

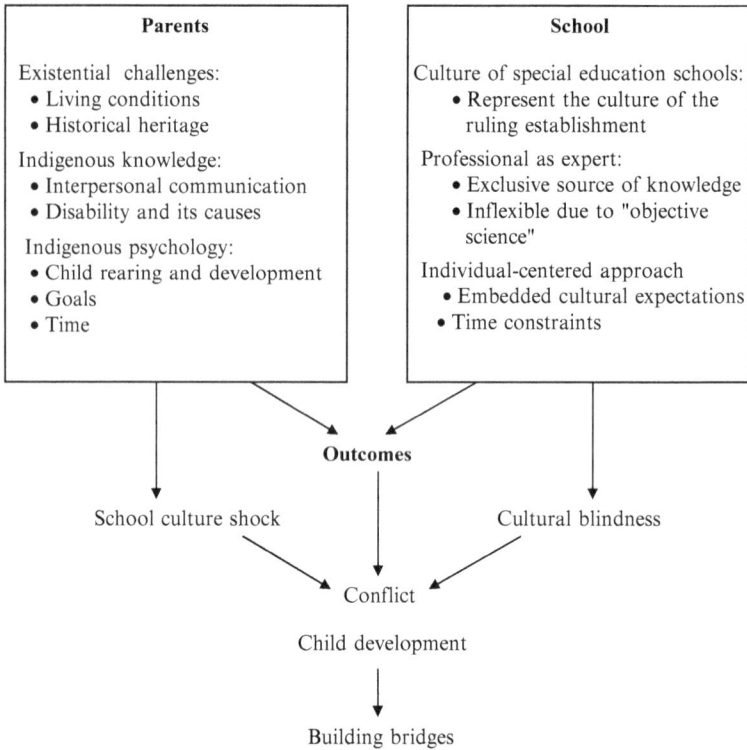

Parents	School

Existential challenges:
• Living conditions
• Historical heritage
 	
Indigenous knowledge:
• Interpersonal communication
• Disability and its causes
 	
Indigenous psychology:
• Child rearing and development
• Goals
• Time
	Culture of special education schools:
	• Represent the culture of the
	  ruling establishment
	
	Professional as expert:
	• Exclusive source of knowledge
	• Inflexible due to "objective
	  science"
	
	Individual-centered approach
	• Embedded cultural expectations
	• Time constraints

Outcomes

School culture shock   Cultural blindness

Conflict

Child development

Building bridges

Fig. 4.4 The dynamic created by the issues and factors that affect collaboration between parents of children with disabilities in indigenous communities and professionals working in special education schools

or insufficient collaboration, might stunt the child's development or certain aspects development. Manifestations of stunted development appear and have an adverse effect in academic; behavioral; emotional; functional; and social aspects of the child's life. The result is that the quality of the child's life either in the present in the future as an adult, is damaged.

I conclude this chapter by presenting a figure that gives a visual representation of the alignment of the issues and factors that were described throughout the chapter, and the manner in which they can lead to the outcomes discussed in the chapter (Fig. 4.4).

Two complementary cultures operate to fulfill the needs of children with disability: one is the indigenous adaptive culture and the other is the public special education school that was established nationally with options for local implementation. The indigenous culture was in existence long before the school, but has not been recognized as such. In order to consider the work being done with the child, it is the task of the professionals to bridge these two cultures.

How, then, does one build a bridge between two cultures? This question has two answers which are in themselves intertwined. The first answer would attempt to attain an understanding of the nature of the differences, by means of academic research examining the different conceptions that each of the parties have on the subject of collaboration between them. The next chapter presents a study that followed this model. The second answer would opt to learn from the results of previous studies conducted in indigenous communities. The last chapter of this book presents studies that follow the second model. I will focus on recommendations that were based on a study which examined the conceptions that both parents and professionals have regarding the subject of collaboration in a specific indigenous community: the Bedouin community in the Negev desert in Israel.

References

Albrecht, G. L., Seelman, K. D., & Bury, M. (2001). *Handbook of disability studies*. Thousand Oaks: Sage.

Amendt, T. (2008). *Involvement to engagement: Community education practices in a suburban elementary school and an inner-city community school*. Unpublished master's thesis, University of Saskatchewan, Saskatoon, SK.

Begay, G. R., Roberts, R. N., Weisner, S. T., & Matheson, C. (1999). Indigenous and informal systems of support – Navajo families who have children with disabilities. *Bilingual Review, 1*, 79–94.

Bempechat, J. (1992). The role of parent involvement in children's academic achievement. *School Community Journal, 83*, 85–102.

BigFoot, D. S. (1998). *Cultural considerations. Upon the back of a turtle. A cross-cultural curriculum for federal criminal justice personnel*. Sponsored by the Office for Victims of Crime, Contract # 96-VR-GX-0002 Copyright © CCAN, OUHSC.

Blanche, E. I. (1996). Alma: Coping with culture, poverty, and disability. *The American Journal of Occupational Therapy, 50*, 265–276.

Bloom, L. R. (2001). "I'm poor, I'm single, I'm a mom, and I deserve respect" advocating in schools and with mothers in poverty. *Educational Studies, 32*, 300–316.

Blue-Banning, M., Summers, J. A., Frankland, H. G., Nelson, L. L., & Beegle, G. (2004). Dimensions of family and professional partnerships: Constructive guidelines for collaboration. *Exceptional Children, 70*, 167–184.

Bowers, C. A. (1995). *Educating for an ecologically sustainable culture: Rethinking moral education, creativity, intelligence, and other modern orthodoxies*. Albany, NY: State University of New York Press.

Boyer, E. (1995). *The basic school: A community for learning*. Princeton, NJ: The Carnegie Foundation for the Advancement of Teaching.

Bradshaw, W. (2013). A framework for providing culturally responsive early intervention services. *Young Exceptional Children, 16*(1), 3–15.

Brandon, R. R. (2007). African American parents: Improving connections with their child's educational environment. *Intervention in School and Clinic, 43*, 116–120.

Bullivant, B. M. (1993). Culture: Its nature and meaning for educators. In J. Banks & C. McGee-Banks (Eds.), *Multicultural education: Issues and perspectives* (2nd ed., pp. 29–47). Needham Heights, MA: Allyn & Bacon.

Burchinal, M., Skinner, D., & Reznic, J. S. (2010). European American and African American mothers' beliefs about parenting and disciplining infants: A mixed-method analysis. *Parenting Science and Practice, 10*, 79–96.

Campinha-Bacote, J. (1999). A model and instrument for addressing cultural competence in health care. *Journal of Nursing Education, 38*, 203–207.

Carter, S. (2002). *The impact of parent/family involvement on student outcomes: An annotated bibliography of research from the past decade. IDEAs that work.* U.S. Office of Special Education Programs. CADRE-Consortium for Appriate Dispute Resolution in Special Education.

Chan, S. (1990). Early intervention with culturally diverse families of infants and toddlers with disabilities. *Young Children, 3*(2), 78–87.

Cho, S. J., Singer, G., & Brenner, B. (2003). A comparison of adaptation to childhood disability in Korean immigrant and Korean mothers. *Focus on Autism and Other Developmental Disabilities, 18*(1), 9–20.

Coffey, A., & Atkinson, P. (1996). *Making sense of qualitative data—Complementary strategies.* Thousand Oaks, CA: Sage.

Colombo, M. W. (2006). Building school partnerships with culturally and linguistically diverse families. *Phi Delta Kappan, 88*, 314–318.

Cook, L., & Friend, M. (2010). The state of the art of collaboration on behalf of students with disabilities. *Journal of Educational and Psychological Consultation, 20*, 1–8.

Cox, D. D. (2005). Evidence-based interventions using home-school collaboration. *School Psychology Quarterly, 20*(4), 473–497.

Creswell, J. (2002). *Research design: Qualitative, quantitative, and mixed methods approaches* (3rd ed.). Thousand Oaks, CA: Sage.

Danseco, E. R. (1997). Parental belief on childhood disability: Insights on culture, child development and intervention. *International Journal of Disability, Development and Education, 44*, 41–51.

De Carvalho, M. E. P. (2001). *Rethinking family-school relations: A critique of parental involvement in schooling.* Mahwah, NJ: Lawrence Erlbaum.

Dempsey, I., Foreman, P., Sharma, N., Khanna, D., & Arora, P. (2001). Correlates of parental empowerment in families with a member with a disability in Australia and India. *Developmental Disabilities Bulletin, 29*, 113–131.

Denzin, N. K. (1997). *Integrative ethnography: Ethnographic practices for the 21st century.* Thousand Oaks, CA: Sage.

Diller, J. V. (1999). *Cultural diversity: A primer for the human services.* Boston: Wadsworth.

Drain, C., & Hall, B. (1986). *Culture shock! Indonesia.* Singapore: Times Books International.

Dunst, C. J., & Dempsey, I. (2007). Family-professional partnerships and parenting competence, confidence, and enjoyment. *International Journal of Disability, Development and Education, 54*(3), 305–318.

Edgerton, R. B. (1970). Mental retardation in non-Western societies: Toward a cross-cultural perspective on incompetence. In H. C. Haywood (Ed.), *Sociocultural aspects of mental retardation* (pp. 523–559). New York, NY: Appleton Century-Crofts.

Epstein, J. (1993). Make parents your partners. *Instructor, 19*, 119–136.

Epstein, J. L. (1995). School, family, community partnerships: Caring for the children we share. *Phi Delta Kappan, 76*(3), 701–713.

Epstein, J. L. (1996). Advances in family, community, and school partnerships. *New Schools, New Communities, 12*(3), 5–13.

Fadiman, A. (1997). *The spirit catches you and you fall down: A Hmong child, her American doctors, and the collision of two cultures.* New York: Farrar, Strauss, & Giroux.

Fine, M. J., & Nissenbaum, M. S. (2000). The child with disabilities and the family: Implications for professionals. In M. J. Fine & R. L. Simpson (Eds.), *Collaboration with parent and families of children and youth with exceptionalities* (pp. 3–26). Austin, TX: Pro-Ed.

Fong, R., Boyd, C., & Browne, C. (1999). The Ghandi technique: A biculturalization approach for empowering Asian and Pacific Islander families. *Journal of Multicultural Social Work, 7*, 95–110.

Frankland, H. C., Turnbull, A. P., & Blackmountain, L. (2004). An exploration of the self-determination construct and disability as it relates to the Dine (Navajo) culture. *Education and Training in Developmental Disabilities, 9*(3), 191–205.

Freire, P. (1970). *Pedagogy of the oppressed.* New York: Herder and Herder.

Friend, M., & Cook, L. (2009). *Interactions: Collaboration skills for school professionals* (6th ed.). Boston: Allyn and Bacon.

Garcia, S. B., Mendez, P, A., & Ortiz, A. (2000). Mexican American mothers' beliefs about disabilities: Implications for early childhood intervention. *Remedial and Special Education, 21*, 90–100, 120.

Goffman, E. (1959). *The presentation of self in everyday life*. New York: Doubleday.

Hanson, M. J., Lynch, E. W., & Wayman, K. I. (1990). Honoring the cultural diversity of families when gathering data. *Topics in Early Childhood Special Education, 10*, 112–131.

Harry, B. (1992). Making sense of disability: Low-income, Puerto Rican parents' theories of the problem. *Exceptional Children, 59*, 27–40.

Harry, B. (2008). Collaboration with culturally and linguistically diverse families: Ideal versus reality. *Exceptional Children, 74*, 373–388.

Harry, B., Hart, J., & Klingner, J. K. (2005). African American families under fire: Ethnographic views of family strengths. *Remedial and Special Education, 26*(2), 101–112.

Harry, B., & Klinger, J. K. (2006). *Why are so many minority students in special education? Understanding race and disability in schools*. New York: Teachers College Press.

Hedeen, T., Moses, P., & Marshall, P. (2011). *Encouraging meaningful parent/educator collaboration: A review of recent literature*. Eugene, OR: Center for Appropriate Dispute Resolution in Special Education (CADRE).

Henderson, A. T., & Mapp, K. L. (2002). *A new wave of evidence: The impact of school, family, and community connections on student achievement. Annual synthesis report*. Austin, TX: National Center for Family and Community Connections with Schools.

Hieneman, M., & Dunlap, G. (2000). Factors affecting the outcomes of community-based behavioral support: Identification and description of factor categories. *Journal of Positive Behavior Interventions, 2*, 161–169.

Kalyanpur, M., & Harry, B. (1999). *Culture in special education: Building reciprocal family-professional relationships*. Baltimore: Paul H. Brookes.

Kalyanpur, M., & Harry, B. (2012). *Cultural reciprocity in special education—Building family-professional relationships*. Baltimore: Paul Brookes.

Kalyanpur, M., & Rao, S. S. (1991). Empowering low-income black families of handicapped children. *American Journal of Orthopsychiatry, 61*, 523–532.

Kasahara, M., & Turnbull, A. P. (2005). Meaning of family-professional partnership: Japanese mothers' perspectives. *Exceptional Children, 71*(3), 249–265.

Knox, M., Parmenter, T., Atkinson, N., & Yazbeck, M. (2000). Family control: The views of families who have a child with intellectual disability. *Journal of Applied Research in Intellectual Disabilities, 13*, 17–28.

Lai, Y., & Ishiyama, F. I. (2004). Involvement of immigrant Chinese-Canadian mothers of children with disabilities. *Exceptional Children, 71*, 97–108.

Lau, A. S. (2010). Physical discipline in Chinese American immigrant families: An adaptive culture perspective. *Cultural Diversity and Ethnic Minority Psychology, 16*(3), 313–322. doi:10.1037/a0018667.

Learning Disabilities Law. (2003). State of Israel (Hebrew).

Lincoln, Y. S., & Guba, E. G. (1985). *Naturalistic inquiry*. Beverly Hills, CA: Sage.

Lo, L. (2005). Barriers to successful partnerships with Ghinese-speaking parents of children with disabilities in urban schools. *Multiple Voices, 8*(1), 84–95.

Lucyshyn, J. M., Dunlap, G., & Albin, R. W. (Eds.). (2000). *Families and positive behavior support: Addressing problem behavior in family contexts*. Baltimore: Paul Brookes.

Lynch, E. W., & Hanson, M. J. (1998). Steps in the right direction: Implications for interventionists. In E. W. Lynch & M. J. Hanson (Eds.), *Developing cross-cultural competence: A guide for working with young children and their families* (pp. 491–512). Baltimore: Paul Brookes.

Lynch, E. W., & Hanson, M. J. (2004). *Developing cross-cultural competence: A guide for working with children and their families* (3rd ed.). Baltimore: Paul Brookes.

Lynch, E. W., & Stein, R. C. (1987). Parent participation by ethnicity: A comparison of Hispanic, Black, and Anglo families. *Exceptional Children, 54*, 105–111.

Maddock, M. (2002). *Home-school relationships: Understandings of children learning at home.* Unpublished doctoral dissertation, University of Cambridge, Cambridge.

Manning, M. L., & Lee, G. L. (2001). Working with parents—Cultural and linguistic considerations. *Kappa Delta Pi Record, 37,* 160–163.

Manor-Binyamini, I. (2003). Collaboration between interdisciplinary teamwork in a special education school. *Issues in Special Education & Rehabilitation, 18*(1), 61–74. Haifa: AHAVA Publishers (Hebrew).

Manor-Binyamini, I. (2004). Collaboration between interdisciplinary teams and parents in special education schools. *Issues in Special Education & Rehabilitation, 19*(2), 35–51. Haifa: AHAVA Publishers (Hebrew).

Mernis, L., & Leininger, R. (1992). *Recommended practices in the identification, assessment, and provision of special education for culturally and linguistically diverse students.* Springfield: Illinois State Board of Education.

Nachshen, J. S. (2005). Empowerment and families: Building bridges between parent and professionals, theory and research. *Journal of Developmental Disabilities, 11*(1), 67–75.

National Education Association. (2008). *Promoting educators' cultural competence to better serve culturally diverse students.* Retrieved November 9, 2008, from www.nea.org/achievement/images/PB13_CulturalCompetence.pdf

Obiakor, F. E., Schwenn, J. O., & Rotatori, A. F. (Vol. Eds.). (1999). *Advances in special education: Vol. 12. Multicultural education for learners with disabilities.* Stamford, CT: Jai Press.

Patton, M. Q. (2001). *Qualitative evaluation and research methods* (2nd ed.). Newbury Park, CA: Sage.

Pedersen, P. B. (1981). Alternative futures for cross-cultural counseling and psychotherapy. In A. J. Marsella & P. B. Pedersen (Eds.), *Cross-cultural counseling and psychotherapy* (pp. 312–337). New York, NY: Pergamon.

Pichette, E. F., Garrett, M. T., & Kosciulek, J. F. (1999). Cultural identification of American Indians and its impact on rehabilitation services. *Journal of Rehabilitation, 65,* 3–10.

Pinkus, S. (2005). Bridging the gap between policy and practice: Adopting a strategic vision for partnership working in special education. *British Journal of Special Education, 32*(4), 174–232.

Rosenfeld, Y. (2002). *Learning from success.* Lecture at the School for the Development of Senior Education Workers in the Education System, Jerusalem.

Sandall, S. P., Smith, B. J., McLean, M. E., & Ramsey, L. (2002). Qualitative research in early intervention/early childhood special education. *Journal of Early Intervention, 25,* 129–136.

Scherzer, A. L. (2009). Experience in Cambodia with the use of a culturally relevant developmental milestone chart for children in low- and middle-income countries. *Journal of Policy and Practice in Intellectual Disabilities, 6*(4), 287–292.

Shannon, K., & Stuart, V. (2005). Helping parents separate the wheat from the chaff: Putting autism treatments to the test. In J. Jacobson, R. M. Foxx, & J. A. Mulick (Eds.), *Controversial therapies for developmental disabilities: Fad, fashion and science in professional practice* (pp. 265–277). Mahwah, NJ: Lawrence Erlbaum.

Skrtic, T. M. (1985). Doing naturalistic research into educational organizations. In Y. S. Lincoln (Ed.), *Organizational theory and inquiry: The paradigm revolution* (pp. 185–220). Beverly Hills, CA: Sage.

Skrtic, T. M. (1991). *Behind special education: A critical analysis of professional culture and school organization.* Denver, CO: Love Publishing.

Skrtic, T. M. (1995). The crisis in professional knowledge. In E. L. Meyen & T. M. Skrtic (Eds.), *Special education and student disability: An introduction: Traditional, emerging, and alternative perspectives* (4th ed., pp. 567–608). Denver: Love Publishing.

Sontag, J. C., & Schacht, R. (1994). An ethnic comparison of parent participation and information needs in early intervention. *Exceptional Children, 60,* 422–433.

Spann, S. J., Kohler, F. W., & Soenken, D. (2003). Examining parents' involvement in and perceptions of special education services: An interview with families in a parent support group. *Focus on Autism and Other Developmental Disabilities, 18*(4), 228–237.

Special Education Law. (1988). The State of Israel (Hebrew).

Stiker, H. J. (1999). *A history of disability* (W. Sayers, Trans.). Ann Arbor: University of Michigan Press.

Stoner, J. B., Bock, S. J., Thompson, J. R., Angell, M. E., Heyl, B. S., & Crowley, E. (2005). Welcome to our world: Parent perception of interactions between parents of young children with ASD and education professionals. *Focus on Autism and Other Developmental Disabilities, 20*(1), 39–51.

Symon, J. B. (2001). Parent education for autism: Issues in providing services at a distance. *Journal of Positive Behavior Interventions, 3*, 160–174.

Te Ahukaramu Charles Royal. (2002). *Indigenous worldviews—A comparative study.* Wellington: Te Wananga-o-Raukawa.

Thomson, G. L. (2003a). Prediction in African American parent: Recommendations to increase the level of parent involvement within African American families. *Journal of Educational Research, 96*, 277–286.

Thomson, G. L. (2003b). No parent left behind: Strengthening ties between educators and African American parents/guardians. *Urban Review, 35*, 7–23.

Turnbull, H. R., Turnbull, A. P., Stowe, M. J., & Huerta, N. E. (2007). *Free appropriate public education: The law and children with disabilities* (7th ed., revised printing). Denver: Love Publishing.

Westerman T., & Wettinfer, M. (1997). *Psychological assessment and intervention of aboriginal people. Psychologically speaking.* Western Australian Psychological Society.

Williams, V., & Robinson, C. (2001). More than one wavelength: Identifying, understanding and resolving conflicts of interest between people with intellectual disabilities and their families. *Journal of Applied Research in Intellectual Disabilities, 14*, 30–46.

Yan, W., & Lin, Q. (2005). Parent involvement and mathematics achievement: Contrast across racial and ethnic groups. *Journal of Educational Research, 99*, 116–127.

Yin, R. (1991). *Case-study research, design and methods* (9th ed.). London: Sage.

Zhang, C., & Bennett, T. (2003). Facilitating the meaningful participation of culturally and linguistically diverse families in the IFSP and IEP process. *Focus on Autism and Other Developmental Disabilities, 18*(1), 51–59.

Part II
Case Study of the Bedouin Community

Chapter 5
Background on the Bedouin Community in Israel

5.1 Background and Characteristics of the Bedouin-Arab Community

Bedouin-Arab is a general name for all nomadic tribes in the Middle East and North Africa. For both Bedouins and anthropologists, the term refers to a lifestyle and value system, as well as to social status, origin, and organization (Al-Kreneawi 2004). Although they are Moslems, Bedouin-Arabs differ from other Arab populations in the world, because they inhabit deserts. Nevertheless, living in certain climate conditions does not imply a unified, racial, ethnic, or national group with a homogenous way of life. Bedouin-Arab populations reside in Egypt, Jordan, Saudi Arabia, Syria, and Israel (Barakat 1993). The process of urban resettlement of Bedouins is a considerably more complicated process in Israel, as the cultural differences between the Israeli and Bedouin societies is greater than that found in other Middle Eastern countries. The Bedouin communities currently residing in the Negev live in the midst of a Western culture, with services provided and organized mainly by the Israeli government.

Three different information sources revealed incompatible data concerning the number of Bedouins residing in the Beer-Sheba region in 2007. According to the Central Bureau of Statistics and the Ministry of Interior, there were 190,000 Bedouins in the Negev that year. Data provided by the Central Bureau of Statistics and the Regional Council of Unrecognized Villages indicated 129,000 Bedouins (Statistical yearbook of the Bedouin in the Negev 2004), half of whom reside in seven urban towns established by the government of Israel: Rahat, Tel-Sheva, Kseifa, Arara, Segev Shalom, Laqiya, and Hura. The other members of the community live in unrecognized villages, known as the "Pzura" (scattered dwellings). The unrecognized villages suffer from a lack of basic services and infrastructure, and they receive very few services from the state.

The Bedouins have retained their language (a Bedouin dialect of Arabic), their religion (Islam), and their social, cultural, economic, and political characteristics.

I. Manor-Binyamini, *School-Parent Collaborations in Indigenous Communities:*
Providing Services for Children with Disabilities, DOI 10.1007/978-1-4614-8984-9_5,
© Springer Science+Business Media New York 2014

Like other indigenous peoples, the Bedouins live as citizens of a nation-state, but as an ethnic majority, they do not belong to the "nation."

The Bedouin culture has specific characteristics; one of these is tribal cohesion—*asabiyya*—which is based on both blood and symbiotic ties that highlight the significance of *nasab* (kinship ties) (Dhaouadi 1990). Another characteristic is that of simplicity, as the Bedouin lifestyle is considered synonymous with naturalness, austerity, and the dignified control over desire in public situations (Barakat 1993).

Al-Krenawi (2000) described the Bedouins in Israel as a "high context" community. It is characterized by a slow pace of societal change and a great sense of social stability, a society in which the collective is emphasized over the individual. Its social structure is patriarchal, which means that a hierarchical order is maintained on the basis of dominance of the male over the female and the older over the younger. The father, a dominant and charismatic figure, is the head of the family: all family members are subordinate to him and respectful towards him. He possesses the legitimate authority to make decisions in every domain of their lives. The individual's interests, therefore, are subsumed under those of the group: the individual maintains allegiance to the group, and follows the community's basic tenet, i.e., the general good of the collective supersedes personal desires. Issues are constructed in the context of the group, not the individual, and thus group members are drawn together in common pursuit of group activities. Likewise, major life decisions such as marriage, where to live, or the range of acceptable occupations are all determined with strong reference to, or often by, the collective. Family members have commitments to each other, even if there is a dispute or disagreement among them, which underscores the Arab proverb: "blood never becomes water." However, if the family has a dispute with an outsider, nothing must take priority over collective bonding in support of the family. This means that each individual lives in an interdependent relationship within the family, viewing himself or herself as an extension of a collective core identity.

The roles and social class of the individual in the tribal Bedouin community vary, depending on one's age and gender. From childhood, a different social path is set for men and women, and there is a clear division of roles on every organizational level. The women are considered of lower standing than the men, but women's standing is also subject to change over the course of their lives, and the different roles they must fulfill. Their sense of identity, and for the most part, their supportive social networks as well, are built on a tribal basis, and the tribe constitutes an affiliation group (Aharoni 2004).

Another major social institution in the Bedouin community is polygamy, which is found in other Muslim or Arab communities, since according to the Koran, it is permissible to marry as many as four women.

Researchers have found that the polygamist family structure has an effect on the family members, in that it predisposes them to higher degrees of marital conflict, family violence, and disruptions (Elbedour et al. 2003). Studies conducted on this community have shown that polygamous marriages are characterized by higher rates of parental conflict, as well as rivalries between both senior and junior wives and full and half-siblings (Elbedour et al. 2003). Moreover, children who experience extreme marital conflict tend to use aggressive behaviors as a means of problem solving and exhibit hostile patterns of communication (Grych and Fincham 1990).

Beyond the characteristics unique to the Bedouin community in Israel, there are characteristics that this community shares with other indigenous communities around the world, and that is the focus of the following subchapter.

5.2 Characteristics, Challenges, and Difficulties That the Bedouin Community Shares with Other Indigenous Communities

This subchapter presents the characteristics, the challenges, and the difficulties that the Bedouin community in the Negev desert faces. This review is organized according to the topics that were introduced in Chap. 1 as common to all indigenous communities in the world.

Many of the researchers that study the Bedouins agree that the Bedouin community in the Negev desert in Israel is an indigenous community (Lithwick 2004; Al-Krenawi and Graham 2008; Berman 2001; Coates 2004; Yiftachel 2003). In 2008, the Bedouin-Arabs made an appeal to the United Nations Permanent Forum on Indigenous Issues (UNPFII), asking to be accepted under an indigenous community status. In that request, they mentioned the following activities, which distinguish the Bedouins as indigenous people (Negev Coexistence Forum for Civil Equality 2008).

– Seeking self-determination as indigenous people
– Being descendants of tribes that lived in the Negev desert prior to the establishment of the State of Israel
– Cultivating an attachment, based on the tradition of subsistence agriculture, to the grazing lands and pastures, to the wells and the waterholes, to the graves and to the villages of the desert, in which they have been living for generations, well before the establishment of the State of Israel in 1948
– Practicing the language, laws, culture, belief system, and customs, which—although based on those of the Arab-Muslim peoples—are unique to them
– Abiding by a social system that is based on tribal affiliation in the context of their grazing areas, known as "the *dira*," and in many cases preserving a traditional economy
– Taking civil, political, and juridical action in order to retrieve lands that belong to them under traditional law

These determinants correspond with various UN definitions (also see Chap. 1 of this book).

5.2.1 High Frequency of Health Risks

A research team working for the organization "Physicians for Human Rights" (with The Regional Council for the Unrecognized Villages in the Negev—RCUV 2012) paints a bleak picture of the health services available in the unrecognized villages in the Negev desert: there is an egregious shortage of both clinics and family health centers, a notable lack of accessibility to the few health services available to the population in the unrecognized villages, and an obvious incompatibility between the needs of the community and the type of services offered. This deficiency is expressed through several prominent phenomena, such as a high infant mortality rate. In 2005, the infant mortality rate among the Arab population in the Negev was 15:1,000, while in the Jewish population the rate was 4.6:1,000 live births. Other indications of poor health status include low life expectancy, as well as a high rate of deficiencies, aberrations, and birth defects. The population also suffers from a high birthrate, environmental infections, and high exposure to trauma. Additionally, 9 % of all Bedouin children in the Negev desert suffer from stunted development, 5 % are underweight, and at 6 months of age, half of the Bedouin children suffer from anemia. Later on, they also develop zinc deficiency, as well as vitamin A and vitamin E deficiency.

Another aspect of life that is recognized as common to indigenous communities throughout the world is an elevated rate of school dropout.

5.2.2   Elevated School Dropout Rates

Due to geographic, linguistic, and religious differences, there is a separate education sector for the Arab population, including the Bedouins. While such separation is legitimate under international law, the disparate amount of resources the Bedouins' schools receive is a clear violation of their rights (Human Rights Watch 2001). In 1998, a special Investigatory Committee on the Bedouin Educational System in the Negev submitted report, at the request of the Minister of Education, to the Ministry's General Director. The committee's main recommendation was that Bedouin education should receive equitable material and human resources—modern facilities, a full range of educational services, special programs, identification of gifted and disabled children, and provision of appropriate programs for them. Thus, the government was called upon to:

• Recognize the needs of unrecognized settlements and build facilities
• Train and increase the number of qualified teachers
• Provide free preschool education for children aged 3–4
• Develop and implement programs for parents
• Address the dropout issue (consider separate education for girls and boys and hire truant officers, school counselors, and social workers)
• Update curriculum and textbooks, making them more relevant
• Institute special enrichment programs
• Provide technical and agricultural education
• Enhance parental involvement
• Include Bedouin educators and community leaders in the southern district Bedouin Educational Authority

The effects that this blatant discrimination has had on the Negev Bedouins are measureable: Bedouins have the highest school-dropout rate in the country (37 %) and the lowest scores on their matriculation examinations (Ministry of Education and Culture 2004). Bedouins who were resettled in the recognized townships, since the late 1960s and onwards, were assigned to the schools in their localities. However, as mentioned, these schools suffer from classroom shortages, poor maintenance, and a general lack of facilities (Human Rights Watch 2001).

The situation for Bedouins living in the unrecognized villages is even worse. The children living in these areas are served by 16 "temporary" elementary schools, located in tin, wooden, or cement buildings (which in most cases are not connected to water or electricity). There is not one high school serving these localities. Due to the lack of infrastructure, children have to travel great distances—on unpaved roads—to reach the schools. This is one of the reasons many Bedouin children do not attend school regularly and, as a result, the number of educated men and women in the Bedouin community in the Negev is significantly low. Another contributing factor is the fact that, traditionally, education has never been in a high priority for them: leading a nomadic life, Bedouins have had to develop skills more suitable to their lifestyle, namely skills that enable survival in the desert (Meir and Barnea 1986). The education of girls and women in particular was viewed as socially insignificant, as women are mainly expected to fulfill the roles of mother and wife.

Despite this, in the area of education, a salient process of improvement has been noted, manifested in an increase in school enrollment rates from one generation to the next, and especially among Bedouin women. While there remains a gap between enrollment rates of men and women, this gap has begun to contract due to women's increased enrollment rates. Primary and junior high school education among the Arab population in Israel has undergone substantial changes in recent decades. Literacy, which 3 decades ago was the privilege of few, has quickly become available to almost all Arab children and youths. In fact, the greatest leap in this respect is seen among the Bedouin communities. The chief improvement has been the increased rate of school attendance in elementary and junior-high schools; however, at higher levels of education, the school attendance rates have remained low, especially among the Bedouins living in the non-recognized villages (Abu-Bader and Gottlieb 2009).

If up to this point the review has considered enrollment and attendance rates, another salient problem that the Bedouin community faces in the area of education is the dropout rate (about 32 %, a mirror image of the school-enrollment rate) at various education levels. As previously noted, problems are uniformly more severe among Bedouin of the non-recognized villages: in this case, the dropout rate among 20 year olds and younger is over 50 % (Abu-Bader and Gottlieb 2009).

Not unlike the trend noted for school enrollment, generational improvement can be seen by comparing the percent of dropouts in a population group aged 44 and older and that found in a population of rates of 20 year olds and younger (Abu-Bader and Gottlieb 2009). Findings indicate a substantial improvement over the years. The biggest improvement (94 % points) was achieved in the reduction of dropout rates at the level of elementary school among Bedouin women of the non-recognized villages. This success is primarily due to the establishment of elementary schools in a number of these villages. By contrast, the least progress was noted in the dropout ratios of Bedouin women for up to 12 years of schooling—only 36 percentage points, which is not surprising given the inadequate number of high schools in these communities. Furthermore, the great distances between non-recognized villages and the nearest high school and the poor condition of the road-infrastructure certainly make students' access to schools more difficult.

5.2.3 Child Labor

There are no data regarding the issue of child labor among the Bedouin community in the Negev desert; however, there are data regarding the dire need for more extensive support services for the community.

5.2.4 The Need for More Extensive Support Services

For over a decade now, researchers have been emphasizing the need for more support services for the Bedouin community, and focusing on the systemic problems and the policies that thwart any such developments (Morad et al. 2006; Abu-Rabia and Weitzman 2002). Another aspect of this issue is the need to create or improve the medical services available to the Bedouin community, to make them compatible with the cultural principles and the actual needs of this community in particular.

The most immediate need for medical support services exists in the case of the Negev Bedouins living in the unrecognized villages, in particular. This crisis has resulted in an increased rate of illnesses and related fatalities. There are several basic health and sanitation problems in the unrecognized localities. There is no waste management infrastructure and as a result, waste accumulates outside the residents' dwellings. These garbage piles are home to disease-carrying pests, such as mosquitoes, flies, wasps, dogs, snakes, rodents, and cockroaches. Many residents choose to burn their solid waste and because they burn organic and inorganic wastes together, various potent toxic chemicals are released into the air. This causes an elevated prevalence of respiratory diseases in these villages (Almi 2003). These villages also lack a sewage system, and consequently residents have resorted to using cesspits located a short distance from their homes. Another factor in the health crisis affecting the Bedouins living in unrecognized villages is that they are not connected to the water supply. Many residents of these localities suffer from dehydration or stomach infections from using unclean water. Some Bedouins collect their water in storage containers, which they have to refill from water-outlets some distance from their place of residence. Others absorb the cost of connecting to the water supply independently (Almi 2003). The shortage of water supply can prove fatal for the Bedouins residing in the Negev desert. Indeed, records from the nearest hospital(Soroka Medical Center) show that each August, the hottest month of the year, about 16,000 Bedouin children are hospitalized, compared to 5,000 Jewish children, even though the Bedouins are a minority population in the Negev (Almi 2003). The Bedouins living in these unrecognized villages are also denied connection to the national electricity grid. Residents often purchase generators at their own expense, which are operated in the evenings. Many homes do not have refrigerators or most types of electrical devices (Almi 2003). This is particularly problematic for Bedouin women, many of whom are confined to the home with an average of eight children (Almi 2003), and must perform household chores without the help of modern electrical devices.

The outcome of this combination of factors has detrimental effects on the Bedouin population. Bedouins have the highest rate of infant mortality in Israel, a high incidence of respiratory diseases, and a large percentage of Bedouin children are hospitalized each year (Almi 2003). Unfortunately, there are not enough medical clinics to serve this population (fewer than 10 clinics serving 76,000 people). The unrecognized villages have no pharmacies, no medical specialists, and ambulances do not enter them (Almi 2003).

5.2.5   Lack of Financial Resources: Poverty

There is not much information available about the Bedouins' employment sources. Various researchers have occasionally released employment data, which tend to be partial and pertain to one village or a group of villages, but not to the entire population of the Bedouin community in the Negev desert. One of the few sources of information, and probably the most comprehensive one, is study of Abu-Bader and Gottlieb (2009), which examines the socioeconomic situation of the Arab-Bedouin population in the Negev and compares it to that of the general Arab population in Israel. There has been a gradual rise in the incidence of poverty over the last decade. In 2004, 52 % of the population in Bedouin population was under the national poverty line, and of this group, nearly two-thirds were persistently poor. By virtue of a unique database of digital mappings, it was possible to learn for the first time about the dire socioeconomic conditions of the Arab-Bedouin population in the unrecognized villages. In the same year (2004), the poverty incidence there was nearly 80 % and its severity was about seven times higher than that prevailing in the secular Jewish society. The findings of that study, which were similar to those obtained in international poverty research, showed that personal and family traits, such as education, age, family size, employment, and occupation of the head of the household, as well as the number of income earners in the family, are important determinants of poverty among the Bedouin population.

The same study also found a significant discrimination in a household's access to basic, infrastructure-related public services. The Bedouin communities' access to infrastructure, especially in non-recognized villages, was so low that it acted as a significant barrier to women's participation in the labor force, thus reducing the number of income earners in the household. The deficient access to infrastructure was also found to have an adverse effect on the completion of studies in schools, and thus indirectly affecting the mothers' childbirth decisions. This deficiency, which impedes investment in human capital, has countered the socioeconomic leverage gained by the education of women.

The socioeconomic situation of the Bedouin population is rife with obstacles, difficulties, and challenges: the rate of unemployment is high; the employment ratio, as a share of the population at working age, is low; and the percentage of school dropouts among children and youngsters insubstantial. This, as well as other factors described in the next section, cause severe and persistent. The share of families with more than seven persons is significantly higher among the Bedouin of the South, as compared to the three other groups (Christians, Druze, and non-Bedouin Muslims). Thus, for example, nearly all families with more than nine persons are Bedouin.

As is the case in other indigenous communities, the lack of financial resources and the resulting poverty are connected also to a history of subjection to acts of dispossession.

5.2.6 Subjection to Acts of Dispossession

The main axis around which the Bedouin community in the Negev desert has been waging long-standing and bitter battles is that of land–territory. In order to gain a comprehensive understanding of this battle, I will first present some background on the Bedouins' settlement in the Negev desert, which is located in the southern part of the State of Israel.

The exact date of the beginning of the Bedouins' settlement in the Negev desert is unknown. Some researchers point out that the waves of immigration of the Bedouin tribes from the Arabian Peninsula began around the time of the Muslim conquests in the seventh century. This migratory trend had several goals: to join the conquering Muslim armies, to search for water sources and pastures during years of drought, and to escape blood vendettas. Entering and settling in the Negev desert happened mainly between the thirteenth to the eighteenth centuries. The Sinai Peninsula and Transjordan became the battlegrounds of feuding tribes that occupied territories and built settlements (Bailey 1980, 1985). The Bedouin community is a layered community, i.e., in addition to the early Bedouin migrants who came from the Arabian Peninsula, in the nineteenth and twentieth centuries; migrant farmers and villagers from the regions of Egypt and the West Bank joined the existing Bedouin community in the Negev. Some of those who joined the community were sharecroppers who worked the lands owned by the Bedouins. Another group comprised migrants from the Sudan who were made to serve as slaves of the Bedouins. Their standing within the Bedouin community is still low to this day (Ben-David 1996).

Researchers investigating the Bedouin society in the Negev desert have noted that the Bedouins are a seminomadic people, and that in their culture and way of life, they attribute great importance to *territory* (Ashkenazi 2000; Grossman 1991). Research shows that it was during the Ottoman period that the majority of the Bedouins adopted a "seminomadic" lifestyle. For several generations, the Bedouin community integrated into its economy a type of agriculture called dry farming. The practice of this agriculture involved a relative stability in the division of lands among the members of the workforce, a division which was achieved through Ottoman mediation and created defined tribal areas. Every Bedouin tribe created its own territorial living area, called "Dira" or "Blad" where its members would settle, work the land, and herd their sheep. The borders of the Dira were modified only occasionally, e.g., after invasions or wars, which gradually became a less frequent occurrence, until the borders of these territories remained completely fixed, in the nineteenth century. Thus, the internal Bedouin system developed as a seminomadic society. Therefore, the traditional ownership system is based on the multigenerational continuity of the tribes and their attachment to specific locations, since the time of the Ottoman Empire (Yiftachel 2010, p. 10).

The Ottoman rule started its de facto reign over the Negev desert using Tanzimat policies at the end of the nineteenth century. Under this framework of rule enforcement, the borders of the tribes living in the Negev desert were clearly defined, and a decision was made to establish the City of Beer-Sheva as a regional center, from which it would be possible to provide services while maintaining tight supervision and control (Avchi 2009). In Beer-Sheva, they built a mosque, a market place, and a court of law, which recognized the traditional structure of the Bedouin society and operated accordingly (Bar-Zvi 1991). The British mandate, which replaced the Ottoman presence, made improvements on the previous means of rule, and the police and the court worked very hard to make the Bedouins abide by British law. In its earliest days, the British mandate formed tribal courts, where Sheikhs served as judges. The objective was to render judgments according to the Bedouin customs, except in the field of criminal law. This relationship between the government and the Mukhtar meant that the Bedouin community would be subject to that government, which in turn meant order, security, and taxes (Ashkenazi 2000).

The 1947 UN partition plan for the division of Palestine into two lands, one Jewish and one Arab, left large parts of the Negev desert outside the borders of the Jewish State, but those were reoccupied in 1948, and included in the Armistice Agreement, and in 1949, declared to be a part of the State of Israel. On the eve of the establishment of the State of Israel, there were 65,000–100,000 Bedouins living in the Negev desert; however, during Israel's War of Independence, the majority of the Bedouins fled or were expelled into Jordan or Gaza and they were not allowed to return at the end of the war. Thus, by the end of the War, there were only 11,000 Bedouins still living in the Negev desert. Prior to the 1948 War of Independence, there were about seven staffs, which contained a hundred tribes, living in the Negev desert, but after 1948, there was only one staff and 17 tribes (Ben-David 1996). These 17 tribes were relocated to the Northwestern part of the Negev desert, which became known as "the Siyagh" (the permitted area). Between the years 1948 and 1966, the Bedouins lived under military rule in the Siyagh area; during that period, the border of the new State cut them off from areas with which they had formerly maintained reciprocal relations. As a result, the Bedouins lived as an isolated minority, separated from their membership group and its social–cultural–economic ties, devoid of political power; refugees who had lost the lands that were once the source of their livelihood (Amiran et al. 1979). From 1948 until the present day, the State of Israel claims that the lands of the Negev desert belong to the State, and that the Bedouins have no rights of ownership. In 1962, a recommendation was made to establish permanent settlements for the Bedouin community, in order to put an end to the Bedouins' claims to land ownership rights, and in 1965, the first Bedouin town in the Negev desert, Tel-Sheva (Tel as-Sabi), was established. By 1989, six more Bedouin towns and villages were established: Rahat, Lakiya, Hura, Kuseife, Shaqib al-Salam (Segev Shalom), and Ar'arat an-Naqab (Ar'ara). These became "recognized villages," but about 50 % of the Bedouin population continued to live outside of these towns, in "unrecognized villages." In 2004, the government authorized 12 more villages to be officially recognized as members of the Abu Basma Regional Council (Yiftachel 2009).

In the case of the Bedouins, much like that of indigenous people in other countries around the world (see Chap. 2), the subject of land and territory emerges as the main axis around which the most bitter and long-standing battles are waged. All countries have difficulty letting go of land and resources, especially if it is of an extensive area. Deprived of both access to the lands and permission to use natural resources, the indigenous community loses its essence and its identity. Not only does the territorial demarcation have economic and cultural implications, it also has political implications, as these peoples are denied the right to self-determination, an issue which makes it even more difficult for countries that espouse the liberal approach and thus are concerned that Bedouins might lose control and supervision rights over the whole area (Tzfadia and Roded 2010).

Table 5.1 reviews the relations between the Government and the Bedouin communities over the year, emphasizing governmental actions that reflect the degree to which the State of Israel recognizes the indigenous community and the type of regime it has maintained over the years in relation to the Bedouins. The review is based on an interpretive analysis of the strategies and practices that have shaped the State's policy in regard to the issue of land. The information in Table 5.1 reveals the deep contradictions that can be found in the existing policies towards the Bedouins.

In regard to the issue of recognition, there is a notable gap between the case of the Bedouins in Israel, in this contemporary, global age, and cases of indigenous groups in other countries. Israel, for most of the characteristics of its policies, is still settled in the Hostile and Indifferent types of recognition. The status and a brief history of some of the indigenous communities in Australia, Canada, and Brazil were outlined in Chap. 2 (see Tables 2.3 and 2.4). Therefore, after presenting the current case of Israel's approach to the Bedouins (Table 5.1), the subsequent Table 5.2, will add to the information presented in Chap. 2, by comparing the treatment of the Bedouins in Israel with Australia's, Canada's, and Brazil's treatment of their indigenous communities.

Tzfadia and Roded (2010) noted that in light of these practices, and their ratings as shown in this Table, it is possible to speak of two primary types of recognition: *hostile recognition* and *indifferent recognition*, both of which correspond to an ethnocratic regime that practices colonialism. This regime typically fluctuates between a growing emphasis on ethnicity and a wish to appear democratic and

Table 5.1 A comparison between the treatment of the Bedouins in Israel with Australia's, Canada's, and Brazil's treatment of their indigenous communities

Regime	Types of recognition	Types of policy	State-indigenous relations
Colonialism	No recognition	– Expansion	1948–1953: expulsion, dispossession, and concentration in Siyagh under military rule
		– Takeover	Later on—militarist treatment: the army—firing ranges, planning military, and police training camps
	Until present day, protective recognition	– Exploitation	Judaization of the region, at present day: 125 Jewish municipalities
		– Oppression	Continuing encroachment and concentration: planning of Bedouin towns and villages since the 1960s
		– Segregation	No recognition of land ownership rights/ demolition of homes and villages
		– Supervision over recognition of uniqueness	Establishment of a supervising body: The Bedouin Directory
	"Protective" recognition	– Segregation	Citizenship and limited rights
		– Oversight, patronage, and limitation of rights	
Ethnocracy	Hostile recognition— until today	– Spatial inequality in allocation of resources creates ethnic-class stratification	– Spatial inequality and discrimination in terms of resource allocation, services, infrastructure, and employment
		– Partial civil rights	– Demolition of homes, spraying of fields, confiscation of herds
		– Spatial encroachment	– Formal civil rights, but in fact no choice as to form of residence, unfair and inclusive planning
		– Economic, social, cultural discrimination	– Planning roads and towns on disputed lands and no resolution on existing towns
		– Declaration of recognition without implementation	– Discourse of expansion and threat
		– Utilization of informal recognition practices	– In unrecognized villages there are no formal addresses, no local government or right to vote, no adequate infrastructure or services
	Indifferent recognition	– Mechanisms of discrimination and inequality	– Plans and announcements
		– Rhetorical recognition	– Unimplemented recommendations of the Goldberg commission
	Until present day	– A passive recognition which does not recognize the special needs of a group with a hostile-confirming type of recognition	– Very little consideration towards the special needs of the community – Giving in to the rulings of the supreme court: providing services, Some recognition for the council of unrecognized villages

(continued)

Table 5.1 (continued)

Regime	Types of recognition	Types of policy	State-indigenous relations
Liberal democracy	The beginnings of affirmative recognition	– Equalizing social and economic conditions	– Establishing shared industrial areas and employment centers in cities
		– Political representation on a liberal basis	– Establishing services and welfare centers
		– Supreme court rulings that promote recognition	– In 2000, recognizing the Abu Basma towns and villages
		– The development of an affirmative legislative agenda	– In 2003, establishing a Regional Council
		– The planning and development of a transformative budget	– One Bedouin member of Knesset
		– Apology and reconciliation	– Establishing an implementation committee and an executive body to implement the recommendations of the Goldberg commission
			– Partial implementation of the recommendations of the Goldberg commission

Adopted from Tzfadia and Roded (2010, p. 139)

open. At the same time, there is a clear trend towards a transformative type of recognition, which is democratic in nature.

As shown in Table 5.2, the land policies of these countries represent an array of different types of recognition. However, in each country, we can find an assemblage of criteria centered around one primary type of recognition, which, in turn, delineates the type of regime. In light of this, we can say that in Canada, the primary type of recognition is an affirmative one, which signifies a democratic, multicultural regime. In Australia, practices revolve around a transformative type of recognition, indicating a mostly liberal and democratic regime. In Brazil, the primary type of recognition is a hostile-confirming one, which suggests that Brazil is undergoing a process of democratization, with alternating trends of progress and regression. Finally, we can see that Israel has fluctuated between hostile and an indifferent recognition.

Gradually there are signs that Israel is moving towards a transformative type of recognition. Thus, for example, the State of Israel is making an effort to address and regularize the recognition issue. Since the establishment of the State of Israel and until present day, Israel has established about 40 committees to address "the problems of the Bedouins." Between the years 1996 and 2000 alone, five committees or interdisciplinary teams were established and authorized to submit recommendation and formulate comprehensive policies to address the Bedouin sector. None of the committees was able to achieve that goal, due to bureaucratic foot-dragging and lack of funding (Committee report regarding the regulation of Bedouin settlement in the Negev and led by Committee Chairman, Retired Judge Eliezer Goldberg 2008).

Table 5.2 Comparison of four countries' treatment of their indigenous populations: Brazil Australia, Canada, and Israel

Country/criterion	Brazil	Australia	Canada	Israel
Colonial background	Spanish occupation in the fifteenth century: 500 years of domination and annihilation	British occupation and settlement imposed at the end of the eighteenth century: 90 % of aboriginals wiped out	Conquests and settlement beginning in the seventeenth century. Independence from the British in 1867	Ottoman and British occupation since the sixteenth century: a lax rule, which allows for a traditional lifestyle
Civil status	Protégés until 1988	Civil status only since 1948. Referendum in 1967 on constitutional amendment granting civil rights 1975—Law forbidding discrimination and allowing for separate governance	Murder, dispossession of livelihood and land since 1876. Native American Act annulled in 1985. Right to vote granted in 1960	Expulsion and dispossession 1948–1953; military rule between 1948 and 1966; receive Israeli citizenship in 1951, which affords them access to services and budgets. Spatial encroachment
Political representation	One representative elected in 1983	One representative in parliament, representation in states	Most representation is in the indigenous organization; underrepresentation in parliament	One member of Knesset, and mayors
Social and economic situation of indigenous peoples	Indigenous rights are violated, forests cleared, hostile army, invasion, plagues, murder, illegalities. Life expectancy dropped from 48 to 42 in a decade; rash of suicides. 60–80 % have chronic disease; child mortality—13 %	Represent the weak in society by a wide margin: poverty, unemployment, crime, alcoholism, disease, and family violence	Indigenous population is younger, less educated, less employed, and earn about 8,000$ less than non-indigenous. Many do not participate in the work force, crime is rampant	A very young Bedouin population (up to 70 % under the age of 18), less educated, lower employment rate than the Jewish population, high unemployment and welfare rates, worse health rates, and higher crime rates
Legal system	Civil law is German 1988-constitution No access to a protective legal framework; indigenous matters are directly subordinate to the federation	Customary+ verbal testimony granting indigenous rights to the land Constitution promoting indigenous status Indigenous matters are directly subordinate to the federation	Customary+ indigenous law No access to a protective legal framework; indigenous matters are directly subordinate to the federation	Customary+Ottoman and British laws. No constitution, law and rulings don't recognize indigenous land rights; supervising body is the Bedouin Directory

(continued)

Table 5.2 (continued)

Country/criterion	Brazil	Australia	Canada	Israel
Land policy	1988 constitution—12 % of State's lands recognized as indigenous land; since then, process of delineation	Crown lands declared terra nullius	1—Legal protection since 1982 and recognition of first rights of indigenous population. Ratified in Constitution Act of 35 (1)	1984—Negev lands are indigenous *Mewat—Halima* "beyond the letter of the law"
	Order No. 1755—encroaches upon indigenous lands	Mabo ruling recognizes indigenous land titles	2—Agreements between tribal leaders and the government	Land rights are unrecognized: official claims can be registered, but the State attempts to nullify them
	87 % of indigenous land ratified in 1993	In 1993—Native Title Act (NTA) ratified and indigenous land tribunal established 1996 decision addresses conflicts and leads to Indigenous Land Use Agreements (ILUAs) NTA ILUA Since 1993, only a few ownership claims have been accepted	3—In 1998, agreement signed for retreat from 750 square miles	recognition of 24 municipalities, yet dozens of villages remain unrecognized with no regularization; discriminatory regularization—suggestions
Data about withheld land	10/93 87 % of land sealed. 11.13 % of land given to half of the population	15 % of the disputed land is defined as indigenous; 2.1 % of the population is given rights to the land	Indigenous make up 5.24 % of the population and 13 % of the disputed land is registered in their name	Bedouins claim 600,000 dunams. The majority of the settled areas are unrecognized, except for the areas of about 20 towns and villages
Self-government	None	Almost no autonomy. From a representative political body in government to regional decentralization	Autonomous existence. 1999 Inuit 1997 Delgamuukw vs. British Columbia and more	None, except for local municipal government
Conflict level	High	Moderate-low	Low	High, though mostly nonviolent
Primary recognition	Hostile-confirming	Affirmative	Transformative	Between hostile and the beginning of transformative

Adopted from Tzfadia and Roded (2010, p. 142)

To conclude this chapter, it is important to emphasize that a review of the past 50 years shows that the Bedouin society in the Negev has undergone significant changes and transformations (Ben-David 1993: Fenster 1995, 1999: Pessate-Schubert 2005), first and foremost, the transition from a traditional, nomadic society to an urban one (Abu-Rabia 2000; Pessate-Schubert 2005) and the rapid absorption of influences related to modernization and globalization. The transition from nomadic life to permanent settlement involved not only changes in dwelling, but also an upheaval in areas of life such as schooling, higher education, the status of women, division of labor, economy, and the labor market (Pessate-Schubert 2005). A society undergoing such a transition must contend with varied challenges. One of these challenges, which will be discussed in the next chapter, is children with disabilities and the special education schools that should accommodate for their needs.

References

Abu-Bader, S., & Gottlieb, G. (2009). *Poverty, education and employment in the Arab-Bedouin society: A comparative view* (Working Papers 98). Jerusalem, Israel: The Van Leer Jerusalem Institute and Social Security Institute. (In Hebrew).

Abu-Rabia, S. (2000). *Different attitudes toward females who drop out of the Bedouin's schools.* M/A thesis, Ben-Gurion University of the Negev, Beer-Sheva, Israel. (In Hebrew).

Abu-Rabia, Y., & Weitzman, S. (2002). Diabetes among Bedouin in the Negev: The transition from a rare to a highly prevalent condition. *Israeli Medical Association Journal, 4*(9), 687–689 (In Hebrew).

Aharoni, R. (2004). Nomads in a modern country: Bedouin in the state of Israel (1948-2004). *Mifne, 25*, 29–35 (In Hebrew).

Al-Krenawi, A. (2000). *Ethno-psychiatry among the Bedouin-Arab of the Negev.* Tel-Aviv, Israel: Hakibbutz Hameuchad House (In Hebrew).

Al-Krenawi, A., & Graham, J. R. (2008). *Helping professional practice with indigenous peoples.* Lanham, MD: University Press of America: Rowman & Littlefield.

Al-Kreneawi, A. (2004). *Awareness and utilization of social, health/mental health services among Bedouin-Arab women, differentiated by type of residence and type of marriage.* Beer-Sheva, Israel: Ben-Gurion University, The Center for Bedouin Studies and Development (In Hebrew).

Almi, O. (2003). *No man's land: Health in the unrecognized villages of the Negev.* Jaffa, Israel: Physicians for Human Rights.

Amiran, D., Shanar, A. E., & Ben-David, I. Y. (1979). The Bedouin settlements in the Be'er-Sheva valley. In A. E. Shmuely & I. Y. Gardos (Eds.), *Land of the Negev: Man and desert* (pp. 652–665). Tel-Aviv, Israel: Ministry of Defense—Publishing House (In Hebrew).

Ashkenazi, T. (2000). *The Bedouin in the land of Israel* (pp. 3–52). Jerusalem, Israel: Ariel Publishing House (In Hebrew).

Avchi, J. (2009). The application of Tanzimat in the desert: The Bedouin and the creation of a new town in southern Palestine (1860-1914). *Middle Eastern Studies, 45*(6), 969–983.

Bailey, C. (1980). The Negev in the nineteenth century: Reconstructing history from Bedouin oral tradition. *Asian and African Studies, 14*(1), 35–80.

Bailey, C. (1985). Dating the arrival of the Bedouin tribes in Sinai and the Negev. *Journal of the Economic and Social History of the Orient, 28*, 20–49.

Barakat, H. (1993). *The Arab world, society, culture, and state.* Berkeley, CA: University of California Press.

Bar-Zvi, S. (1991). *The judicial tradition of the Negev Bedouins*. Tel-Aviv, Israel: Ministry of Defense—Publishing House (In Hebrew).

Ben-David, Y. (1993). *The Bedouin educational system in the Negev: Reality and the need for progress*. Jerusalem, Israel: Florsheimer Institute for Policy Research (In Hebrew).

Ben-David, Y. (1996). *Negev dispute: Bedouins, Jews and land*. Jerusalem, Israel: Center for Arab Studies (In Hebrew).

Berman, G. S. (2001). Social services and indigenous populations in remote areas. *International Social Work, 49*(1), 97–106.

Coates, K. S. (2004). *A global history of indigenous peoples: Struggle and survival*. Houndmills, England: Palgrave Macmillan.

Committee report regarding the regulation of Bedouin settlement in the Negev, led by Committee Chairman, Retired Judge Eliezer Goldberg. (2008). Retrieved from http://www.moch.gov.il/NR/rdonlyres/770ABFE7-868D-4385-BE9A-:96CE4323DD72/5052/DochVaadaShofet GoldbergHebrew3.pdf. (In Hebrew).

Dhaouadi, M. (1990). Ibn-Khaldun: The founding father of Eastern sociology. *International Sociology, 5*(3), 319–335.

Elbedour, S., Onwuegbuzie, A. J., & Alatamin, M. (2003). Behavioral problems and scholastic adjustment among Bedouin-Arab children from polygamous and monogamous marital family structures: Some developmental considerations. *Genetic, Social, and General Psychology Monographs, 129*, 213–237.

Fenster, T. (1995). Planning and development in Bedouin settlements by gender and space. *Mivnim, 158*, 68–83 (In Hrbrew).

Fenster, T. (1999). Space for gender: Cultural roles of the forbidden and the permitted. Environment and planning, D. *Society and Space, 17*, 227–246.

Grossman, D. (1991). The Arab village and its daughters. In D. Grossman & A. Meir (Eds.), *The Arab settlement in the land of Israel—Geographical processes*. Beer Seva, Israel: Ben-Gurion University (In Hebrew).

Grych, J. H., & Fincham, F. D. (1990). Marital conflict and children`s adjustment: A cognitive-contextual framework. *Psychological Bulletin, 108*(2), 267–290.

Human Rights Watch. (2001). *Second class: Discrimination against Palestinian Arab children in Israel's schools*. New York, NY: Author.

Lithwick, H. (2004). *A preliminary evaluation of the negevbedouins experience of urbanization*. Beer-Sheva, Israel: Negev Center for Regional Development (In Hebrew).

Meir, A., & Barnea, D. (1986). *The development of the Bedouin educational system in the Negev*. Southern District, Israel: The Ministry of Education, Culture and Sports (In Hebrew).

Ministry of Education and Culture. (2004). *Matriculation examination data for 2003*. Jerusalem, Israel: Author (In Hebrew).

Morad, M., Shvarts, S., & Merrick, J. (2006). The influence of Israel health insurance law on the Negev Bedouin population—A survey study. *Scientific World Journal, 24*(6), 81–95.

Negev Coexistence Forum for Civil Equality. (2008). *The indigenous Bedouin of the Negev desert in Israel*. Submitted to UN Working Group on Indigenous Populations.

Pessate-Schubert, A. (2005). Retelling her-story: To be a female Bedouin teacher differently. *Comparative Education, 3*, 247–266.

Statistical yearbook of the Bedouin in the Negev. (2004). In cooperation with Konrad Adenauer Foundation. www.kas.de/israel.

The Regional Council for the Unrecognized Villages in the Negev—RCUV. (2012). *Blueprint for recognizing the unrecognized villages in the Negev*. Lakiya, Israel: Sidreh–Lakiya Foundation (A project funded by the European Union) (In Hebrew).

Tzfadia, E., & Roded, B. (2010). *Recognition and indigenous land rights: The case of the Arab-Bedouins in the Negev—A comparative perspective*. Beer-Sheva, Israel: Ben-Gurion University of the Negev, The Robert H. Arnow Center.

Yiftachel, O. (2003). Bedouin-Arabs and the Israeli settler state: Land policies and indigenous resistance. In D. Champagne & I. Abu-Saad (Eds.), *The future of indigenous peoples: Strategies for survival and development* (pp. 21–47). Los Angeles, CA: American Indian Studies Center Publication, UCLA.

Yiftachel, A. E. (2009). Preparing to recognize Bedouin villages? Planning the Be'er-Sheva metropolis in light of the Goldberg commission. *Tichnun, 6*(1), 165–184 (In Hebrew).

Yiftachel, A. E. (2010). *Expert opinion: A response to the opinion of Professor Ruth Kark regarding the claims of the heirs of Suleiman Al-Oqbi for land ownership in Al-Araqib and Zhilika.* Be'er-Sheva, Israel: District Court (In Hebrew).

Chapter 6
Children with Disabilities and Special Education in the Bedouin Community in Israel

6.1 An Overview of Children with Disabilities in the Bedouin Community

In order to present a reliable overview, it is important to know how many children with disabilities there are in this community. Different information sources revealed incompatible data concerning the number of Bedouin children with disabilities in the Negev region. There is a significant gap between the numbers reported by the Department of Welfare Services, The Ministry of Education, and Israel's Social Security Institute, and the actual number of Bedouin children with disabilities in the Negev region. Government organizations do not have accurate information about the population of Bedouin children and youth in the Negev. Thus, for example, if we rely on the data presented in a nationwide survey conducted in 2000 by the Brookdale Institute in collaboration with Israel's Social Security Institute, Children with Special Needs—Evaluation of Needs and their Service Coverage (Naon et al. 2000), it appears that in the Arab (not the Bedouin) sector, the percentage of children with severe disabilities is 4.2 % according to the following distribution: intellectual disability—0.8 %, sensory disabilities (deafness and blindness)—1.4 %, severe physical disabilities (cerebral palsy, spina bifida, skeletal and muscular illness)—2 %.

Extrapolating from statistical data regarding the Arab population in northern Israel, Table 6.1 presents the estimated number of children with disabilities in the Bedouin community in the Negev, by locality.

Furthermore, there is an additional gap between the estimates presented in Table 6.1 and the actual state of affairs in the unrecognized Bedouin villages. Table 6.2 illustrates the difficulty involved in gathering accurate data about the Bedouin community. In a meeting that took place on 15 June 2005, between the Department of Welfare Services and representatives of children with disabilities, the deputy director of the southern region in the Ministry of Social Welfare, who was in charge of the supervision and treatment of children and adults with autism, presented data that did not correspond to the numbers expected based on the percentage of people with autism in the general population. The comparison presented

I. Manor-Binyamini, *School-Parent Collaborations in Indigenous Communities:*
Providing Services for Children with Disabilities, DOI 10.1007/978-1-4614-8984-9_6,
© Springer Science+Business Media New York 2014

Table 6.1 Evaluation of children with disabilities in the Bedouin community in the Negev

Locality	No. of residents	No. of children under 18	Intellectual disability (0.8 %)	Children with sensory disabilities (1.4 %)	Children with physical disabilities (2 %)	Total
			Extrapolation based on data from a nationwide survey conducted by the Brookdale Institute and Israel's Social Security Institute			
Rahat	35,800	22,837	183	320	457	959
Tel-Sheva	11,900	7,500	60	105	150	315
Arara	11,000	6,500	52	91	130	273
Kseifa	8,500	4,800	38	67	96	202
Hura	8,200	4,868	39	68	97	204
Laqiya	6,600	3,300	26	46	66	139
Segev Shalom	5,500	3,200	26	45	64	134
Unrecognized villages	70,000	42,000	336	588	840	1,764
Total	157,500	95,005	760	1,330	1,900	3,990

Adopted from Manor-Binyamini (2007)

Table 6.2 The number of children/adults with autism in comparison with the expected number

Locality	Number of autistic children/youth in the village	Expected (in relation to the percentage in the general population)
Mytar (Jewish)	7	6
Lehavim (Jewish)	4	5
Segev Shalom (Bedouin)	1	5
Laqiya (Bedouin)	1	8
Rahat (Bedouin)	3	35
Data related to Kseifa, Hura, and the unrecognized villages is missing	–	–

in Table 6.2 suggests that there are problems involved in identifying, not to mention treating, children with disabilities in the Bedouin community.

Kesher Organization, a nongovernmental organization that serves families of children with disabilities, presented the following picture in 2011: in the Bedouin community, the percentage of children with disabilities relative to the total number of children in the community was 9.1 %; parallel percentages were 8.3 % in the population of Arab children and 7.6 % in the population of Jewish children (Kesher Organization 2011). The absence of data regarding complex disabilities, whereby a child suffers from more than one primary disability, is especially notable in the Bedouin community. A study on this subject investigated the prevalence and the types of psychiatric disorders found among adolescent Bedouins with mild to moderate intellectual disability. Findings indicated that 77 % of the adolescents had at least one psychiatric disorder during the evaluation, the most common of these were autism-spectrum disorders—70 % (21); disruptive disorders—47 % (14); attention deficit and hyperactivity—47 % (14); and anxiety disorders—40 % (12). Other psychiatric disorders of lower frequency were also found and discussed in the findings (Manor-Binyamini 2010). These results suggest a high rate of complex disabilities.

A reliable summary regarding the conditions of children with disabilities in the Bedouin community should address the reasons for the high rates of children with disabilities in this community. One of the several possible factors that contribute to this phenomenon includes mothers who continue to give birth at an older age. The high incidence of brain damage at birth is often due to premature births, hereditary diseases that cause physical and mental disabilities, and congenital deformities of the skeletal and nervous systems (Dagirmanjian 1996; Israeli Knesset Center for Research and Study 2006). In the Bedouin community, like in North and sub-Saharan Africa, the Middle East, and in West, Central, and South Asia, there is a strong cultural preference for consanguineous marriage; thus, between 20 % and over 50 % of marital unions are intrafamilial, most commonly between first cousins (Bittles 2001). Consanguinity increases the rate of expression of deleterious recessive gene mutations that are associated with disorders such as phenylketoneuria (PKU), Smith–Lemli–Opitz syndrome (SLO), Prader–Willi syndrome, Angelman syndromes, L1 (a neural cell adhesion molecule)-associated conditions, and autosomal recessive microcephaly (Henderson 2004; Muir 2000; Jackson et al. 1998). A study conducted in Beer-Sheva assessed the cognitive and neuropsychological symptoms found among children who had been hospitalized for poisoning before the age of 3 and compared these with the findings of the same assessment conducted in a group of matched controls (Kofman et al. 2004). More than 90 % of the hospitalization cases were of Bedouin children. Results showed that kerosene poisoning impaired verbal memory and, in addition, the poisoned group demonstrated impaired ability to inhibit prepotent behaviors when distracted (Kofman et al. 2004). Furthermore, data from the Ministry of Health point to a high rate of infant mortality and infant hospitalization in the Bedouin sector. This is caused by inappropriate health and safety conditions in the unrecognized Bedouin villages.

In addition to the factors that can explain the high rate of children with disabilities in the Bedouin community, there are certain characteristics of this population that directly affect the quality of life of children with disabilities; the following are the main ones (Manor-Binyamini 2007). The first factor is the acute socio-economic conditions of numerous Bedouin families. Bedouin villages are characterized by lower than average family income, a high rate of unemployment, and little commercial or industrial activity (Lithwick 2002, p. 2). In light of limited sources of income and severe economic hardship, most families, which in most cases have many children, live on child welfare payments; in the case of a disabled child in the family, there are additional disability benefits. There are also severe transportation and accessibility problems, particularly in unrecognized villages. Due to the very limited public transportation that reaches the Bedouin towns and villages, the high cost of alternative transportation services, and the restricted mobility imposed on women, mothers are forced to carry their disabled children several kilometers to the main road and to wait there for a passing car, in order to reach a treatment center. This situation is exacerbated due to the tradition which restricts women's movement to remaining within the confines of their residential area. Hence, every trip she takes from the domain of the tribe mandates accompaniment by a male relative. Consequently, every visit she makes to the a child development clinic or center, which is usually situated in a locality far from her place of domicile, depends on the availability and willingness of her male relatives (The Forum for Advancing Children and Youth with Special Needs in the Bedouin Community 2003). Another contributing factor is the share of large families with many children. Bedouin mothers must care for numerous children and find it difficult to be active partners in the rehabilitation process. In most cases, mothers of children with disabilities must cope alone with the difficulties of raising and caring for these children.

From the professional perspective, one of the characteristics of intervention intended for children with disabilities is that it is a long-term process. Many parents find this to be highly demanding in terms of the continuous and long-term investment that the therapeutic-rehabilitative process requires. Bedouin daily life, which demands immediate solutions to existential problems, does not easily adjust to coping with long-term objectives. Furthermore, data from the Child Development Center at the Soroka Medical Center in Beer Sheba show that a high percentage of Bedouin children with disabilities do not receive proper rehabilitative treatment. Traditional patterns of child rearing are an additional characteristic of Bedouin society, with ramifications for the treatment of children with disabilities. Playing and mediation are the two most important principles of developmental intervention; however, the arduous living conditions and the large number of children leave almost no time for Bedouin mothers to play with their children (The Forum for Advancing Children and Youth with Special Needs in the Bedouin Community 2003).

The particularly arduous environmental conditions are another significant characteristic: the living conditions in unrecognized villages, i.e., huts and tents with irregular electricity and running water, exacerbate the hardships involved in caring for children with special needs and hinder the use of equipment and advanced technology such as wheelchairs, walkers, computers, alternative means of communication, and other aids which can improve the quality of life of the children and their family. An issue currently under discussion in numerous countries pertains to children's rights. Bedouin society is in the process of transitioning from a traditional to a modern society, yet this society still lacks sufficient awareness of children's rights in general and the rights of the child with special needs in particular. The overview presented here points to the fact that children with disabilities are a particularly vulnerable population, in need of support services. This will be the focus of the following section.

6.2   Special Education in the Bedouin Community in Southern Israel's Negev Region

The goal of this section is to present an overview of the special education system available to the Bedouin community; to this end, I will discuss the following issues: physical infrastructure; multidisciplinary professional personnel; insufficient methods and tools for diagnosis, placement, and intervention; and the absence of support services for special education needs.

6.2.1 *Physical Infrastructure*

In 1991, the State Comptroller's annual report indicated that special education schools for children with disabilities from the Bedouin community are virtually nonexistent, posing significant difficulties to those in need of such services. As of 2005, there were only three special education schools in the entire Bedouin sector, located in the towns of Kseifa, Hura, and Rahat.

The table shows that as of 2005, there were no schools for Bedouin children with diverse disabilities, such as autism or behavioral disorders. Not only does the lack of suitable frameworks leave many children without proper care, it is important to note that attending frameworks that are unsuited to their needs may actually be harmful to the children's development. Thus, for example, due to the shortage of settings for children with severe behavioral disturbances, these children might be referred to psychiatric centers, instead of receiving proper care in the community or in a suitable daycare center.

6.2.2 *Multidisciplinary Professional Personnel*

The unique characteristics of the special education school require the collaboration of a multidisciplinary team. According to the Margalit Committee report (Mazawi 1997), only 30 % of all children with disabilities in the Bedouin community in the Negev received the social security disability benefits and paramedical services to which they were entitled, compared to 73 % of the children with disabilities in the Jewish sector. There is a significant shortage of professionals in several fields, most notably in the paramedical professions, such as physical, occupational, and speech therapy. As a result, there are fewer paramedical professionals available to work in the Bedouin schools. It is important to emphasize that without the presence of paramedical professionals on the multidisciplinary teams at the schools, it is impossible to make the necessary adaptations to the curricula for the children with disabilities in the Bedouin sector. In effect, this limits the care they receive, which in turn hinders their development. As a case in point, an insufficient number of qualified diagnosticians impedes necessary diagnostic activities, and, due to a shortage of professionals in treatment fields, the children that are diagnosed do not receive the proper physical/emotional/behavioral treatment. Furthermore, due to a scarcity of support personnel to assist the teaching staff, teachers face greater difficulties in the classroom. Table 6.3 lists the paramedical services available in the Bedouin special education field as of 2005.

To illustrate the problem, I chose to focus on one professional field, that of speech therapy. The speech therapist's role is to diagnose and treat pupils with hearing, communication, language, and/or speech difficulties. Speech therapists work in collaboration with the multidisciplinary team in the educational framework, in accordance with the educational goals defined for each pupil. As part of the treatment process, the speech therapist provides counseling and guidance to the

Table 6.3 Types of paramedical services in special education available in the Bedouin sector for 2005

Types of paramedical services	Per locality
Speech therapists	3
Occupational therapists	1
Physical therapy	2
Art therapists	8

From Abu-Ajaj (2005)

professional team and to the parents, to ensure that work on communication, language, and hearing will be integrated into the pupil's daily routine.

As shown in Table 6.3, speech therapy is one of the fields with the most significant shortage of professionals. In 1998, Professor Ornoy, advisor to the Minister of Health, told the Committee on the Status of the Child that there was a shortage of 259 speech therapists in the Arab education system (Ornoy 1998). This shortage has myriad ramifications resulting in impeded education, rehabilitation, and development of children with special needs. The scarcity of speech therapists in the Arab sector is especially significant, as it hinders the integration of children with special needs into Arab society, since children treated by a speech therapist that is not a native speaker of Arabic do not learn the language of the social environment in which they live.

The Ben-Peretz Committee recognized the shortage of professionals in the Arab special education system and recommended adding 50 professionals who would be especially trained to treat complex disabilities (The Ministry of Education 1998). An extensive search conducted as part of the current research did not produce any documentation indicating implementation of this recommendation.

In the special education school in Israel, the homeroom teacher is the key professional. Homeroom teachers working with children with disabilities fill numerous and varied roles. In light of their specific training, these teachers are responsible for following the child's development, which includes diagnosing the child; conducting an evaluation and providing a profile of the child's strengths and weaknesses; defining educational and treatment goals in accordance with the child's specific needs; preparing an Individual Education Plan (IEP) in collaboration with all of the professionals working with the child; overseeing the implementation of the IEP and the treatment designated by the multidisciplinary team. The homeroom teachers in special education frameworks provide either individualized or group remedial skill-building sessions, with or without the input from an additional professional. Returning to our example, a speech therapist might join the individualized or group session, to incorporate treatment into the learning session and thus track the pupil's progress. In addition to working with the pupils, the homeroom teacher is the point person for the support personnel and for parents, providing information and guidance concerning drilling and reinforcing the study material, and for expanding the educational team's knowledge regarding necessary adjustments within a specific educational environment. As part of the trend towards involving parents in determining appropriate intervention methods and deciding on specific goals and objectives, it is the homeroom teacher's responsibility to work with parents and guide

Table 6.4 Special education teachers according to level of education

	Hebrew education (%)	Arabic education (%)
Academic	55	30
Uncertified	5	14

Lubetzky et al. (2004) and Galil et al. (2001)

them in implementing the decisions and recommendations in the home environment. Homeroom teachers also serve as coordinators among all the entities working with the pupil in the educational school, transmitting information, coordinating approaches, and formulating priorities. The professional responsibilities delineated above require homeroom teachers to receive a broad and high-quality training in the special education field. Furthermore, their strategic role highlights the need for highly competent homeroom teachers, able to successfully fill the myriad roles assigned to them by the special education school system.

Table 6.4 presents data regarding the qualification of special education teachers who, as described by The Ministry of Education, serve as key figures, working with the children, the parents, and the other team members (Lubetzky et al. 2004; Galil et al. 2001).

Morad et al. (2004) found a shortage both of personnel trained in special education with a specialization in teaching children with disabilities and of the associated support services that provide early childhood preventive intervention and parental guidance.

Regarding the support services available to the community, according to a research report by the Brookdale Institute (2008), the percentage of Bedouin children who receive at least one type of support service is much lower than that found in the Jewish sector. According to the data, the percentages of children who receive disability benefits in the Bedouin settlements in the Negev desert, per 1,000 residents are as follows: Rahat—10.6 %, Ar'ara—7.3 %, Hura—9.5 %, Kuseife—10.2 %, Lakiya—8.7 %, Segev Shalom—7.1 %, and Tel-Sheva—12.7 %. The percentages of children who receive disability benefits in other Bedouin settlements of similar size are 20–50 % lower than those in the Jewish sector. Additionally, according to the research report, a comparison between the data for 2005 and the data for 1996 regarding the allocation of services to children with disabilities in the different sectors revealed the following picture: only 2 % of Bedouin parents compared to 14 % of Jewish families of children with disabilities received family counseling, 10 % compared to 8 % received an allowance from social security, 20 % compared to 39 % received paramedical treatment, and 37 % compared to 81 % received at least one type of support service. When comparing recognized villages to unrecognized Bedouin villages, researchers found yet another bleak picture: in recognized villages, 12 % of the children with disabilities received paramedical treatment, compared to 8 % of unrecognized villages; and 44 %—compared to 8 %—received medical treatment, special education, and psycho-social assistance.

6.2.2.1   Insufficient Methods and Tools for Managing the Diagnosis, Placement, and Intervention Programs for Children with Disabilities

Arab diagnostic and therapeutic frameworks in Israel are not equipped, systemically or professionally, to provide children with disabilities equal opportunities for realizing their full-fledged capabilities in their own language, while participating in the cultural and social life of their environment and community. A reference to the issue as it relates to the Bedouin sector can be found in the response of the former Minister of Education, Mr. Yossi Sarid (1999), to a parliamentary question submitted by Arab Knesset Member Mr. Barakkeh. On the one hand, the Minister's reply clearly shows that for many years, Arab students have been overrepresented among children with disabilities. On the other hand, in his response, the Minister noted that only a negligible number of individuals were diagnosed with learning disabilities among Arab students, and that, similarly, very few children among Arab students were diagnosed with autism, psychological disorders, behavioral disorders, language problems, or developmental problems. This underrepresentation is the result of a shortage of diagnostic services as well as diagnostic tools in the Arab sector; the tools and services that are available have not been adapted to the specific needs of this sector. Consequently, many children cannot benefit from the services to which they are entitled. In some cases, due to the absence of a formal diagnosis, children are labeled erroneously and, as a result, they are forced to contend with both social and psychological hardships. Due to insufficient valid and reliable diagnostic tools, in particular, didactic tests adapted to the needs of Arab schools, inadequate diagnosis may lead to alienation and cause social and cultural harm.

The curricula in Arab special education schools are often based on the translation of the corresponding Hebrew curricula. In this regard, it is important to note that the social–cultural context that affects the environment's overall relationship towards children with disabilities is fundamentally different in Jewish and Arab societies. Consequently, translation of an intervention program is—in and of itself—insufficient. There is a need to modify these programs and adapt them to the community and society in which the children with disabilities reside. In 1999, the Ben-Peretz Committee recommended allocating three teaching positions to The Ministry of Education's Curriculum Department; these individuals would be assigned the responsibility of preparing books and learning materials appropriate for the special education population in the Arab sector (The Ministry of Education, Culture and Sports 1998, p. 2). Documentation indicating implementation of this recommendation to date was not found.

6.2.3   Support Services

Analysis of assorted data sources shows that despite the far-reaching needs of the Bedouin population in the Negev, there is a (inverse) gap between the special education support services available to the Jewish and the Bedouin sectors. Only a few prominent examples are reviewed here.

The Regulation for the Safe Transportation for Disabled Children stipulates that the local authority is obliged to provide transportation to and from the educational institution suited to the special needs of children with disabilities, which includes appropriate accompaniment and suitable safety measures. Although obligatory provisions and safety procedures do exist, in the Arab sector these provisions are not enforced in most cases. Consequently, children with disabilities in this sector are at risk for severe physical injury (Shatil Organization for Social Change 2002).

Another area in which there is a noticeable gap between the services available to each sector is that of nongovernmental assistance and resources. In addition to the government of Israel, voluntary organizations are active in the field of special education in general, and with respect to specific populations, in particular. Most of these organizations were established by parents in order to improve the level of educational and rehabilitative services provided to their children. Some organizations receive funds from the government to purchase services. In addition, various support services are available through organizations such as *Akim*—a nonprofit organization for advancing the mentally handicapped, *Alut*—a national organization for autistic children, and *Shema*—an organization for educating and rehabilitating hearing-disabled children. The voluntary and nonprofit organizations provide services that are not supplied, or are only partially supplied, by government entities. Thus, for example, *Micha* provides educational services to hearing-disabled children of ages 0–3 years, who are not entitled to receive services from The Ministry of Education. The majority of organizations play a significant role in increasing public awareness regarding the needs of children with disabilities, and either lead or participate in legal and public efforts that aim at ensuring the rights of children with disabilities. Wisel et al. (2000, p. 15) found that despite the importance of the organizations and nonprofit organizations, they are—for the most part—not active in the Arab sector. Among the active organizations worthy of mention in the Arab sector are *Bizchut*, *Adalah*, and *Shatil*, as well as the Action Committee for Arab Special Education in the Negev. The majority of these organizations are nonprofit organizations, with heavy parental involvement. As such, they constitute a collaborative framework between professionals and parents, enabling the latter to take responsibility, develop leadership, and lead significant change processes. Parental leadership is important because cultural diversity (Turnbull and Turnbull 2001) cannot be realized if families do not participate in the future planning dialog (Callicott 2003).

The findings presented here clearly indicate the need for a comprehensive intervention program aimed at narrowing the gaps and ensuring affirmative action in special education in the Bedouin sector. Affirmative action policies are an imperative, if we wish to provide equal opportunities to children with special needs in the Arab education system, despite the huge gap between the Arab and Jewish educational systems in terms of the rate of available services developed specifically to address special education needs. Through affirmative action we can begin to compensate for the outcomes of economic hardship, endured on a personal level by parents in the Bedouin society, as well as on a systemic level, by Arab local governments and nongovernment organizations, as they all attempt to address the special education needs, both in the Arab sector in general and in the Bedouin society in particular.

Corroboration of the severity of the problems and issues previously described can be garnered from the recommendations proposed by the Margalit Committee (2000, Recommendation b,1).

> The Committee recommends taking affirmative action in allocating resources and developing services for underprivileged social groups in the field of special education in the Arab educa-tion system in general, and in the education system serving Bedouin villages in particular. This affirmative action policy will be reflected in allocating the required resources for devel-oping an infrastructure and for training professional personnel in the relevant spheres, in order to narrow gaps and ensure equality and equity in access to special education services.

In other words, a solution requires the pooling resources and services, the inte-gration of education and rehabilitation services into the framework of the commu-nity, as well as an appropriate framework for children of all ages in order to ensure their continued advancement in all areas of life. An urgent overall systemic effort is also required, in order to develop a qualitative community infrastructure capable of providing a holistic and inclusive response to children with disabilities in the Bedouin community and sector.

To conclude this chapter, I wish to describe the efforts undertaken to address the grim situation outlined herein. In 1999, The Forum for Advancing Children and Youth with Special Needs in the Bedouin Community was established in the Negev desert. The participants in this forum are academics and professionals, Bedouins and Jews, from a variety of fields (education, health, psychology, and social work), as well as a representative of the community. Since its establishment, the Forum has acted to identify the needs of Bedouin children with disabilities, and to help promote high-quality programs in the field of special education. After examining the situation thoroughly, the Forum formulated the idea of a regional campus that would serve as a model of quality and excellence in the field of special education, and serve as a center for practical training and research. The idea was enthusiastically received by The Ministry of Education, and a formal cooperation between the Forum and The Ministry of Education was formed in order to build this campus. According to the plans, this campus is intended to serve 570 children and adolescents, from 18 months to 21 years of age, most of whom reside in the Abu-Basma regional council and in unrecognized villages. The plans also stipu-lated that the campus would include 6 rehabilitative daycare centers, 12 special education kindergartens, 5 special education schools, a center for rehabilitation and health, a sports and recreation center, and an academic unit for practical train-ing. The design stage has been completed. The design shown in Fig. 6.1 represents nearly 6 years of planning and investment by the Forum, intended to improve the conditions of children with disabilities in this sector. The campus is currently under construction.

Simultaneously with the planning of the campus began the process of identifying and training multidisciplinary teams that would work in the planned campus. Training took place at the Department of Education of the Ben-Gurion University of the Negev, between the years 2004 and 2005 (on Planning, implementation and evaluation of training, see Manor-Binyamini 2005).

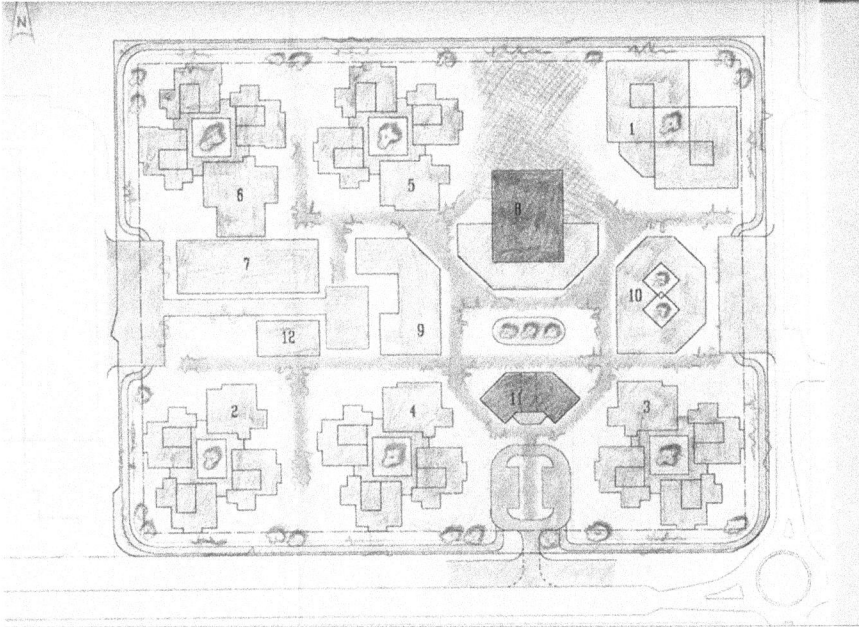

Fig. 6.1 A campus for children with disabilities in the Bedouin community of the Negev desert. *Map Legend*: *1* kindergarten, *2* high school, *3* elementary school, *4* elementary school, *5* school for children with autism, *6* high school, *7* vocational training center, *8* center for sport and arts, *9* dining room, *10* rehabilitation center, and *11* academic centers

References

Abu-Ajaj, A. (2005). *Special education in the Bedouin sector.* Southern Region: Ministry of Education Publishing Company.

Bittles, A. H. (2001). Consanguinity and its relevance to clinical genetics. *Clinical Genetics, 60,* 89–98.

Brookdale Institute. (2008). *Special needs children in the Bedouin community of the Negev desert.* Jerusalem, Israel, Research Report by the Center for Disabilities and Special Populations.

Callicott, K. J. (2003). Culturally sensitive collaboration within person-centered planning. *Focus on Autism and Other Developmental Disabilities, 18,* 60–68.

Dagirmanjian, S. (1996). Armenian families. In M. McGoldrick, J. Giordano, & J. K. Pearce (Eds.), *Ethnicity and family therapy* (pp. 376–391). New York, NY: Guilford.

Galil, A., Carmel, S., Lubetzky, H., Vered, S., & Heiman, N. (2001). Compliance with home rehabilitation therapy by parents of children with disabilities in Jews and Bedouin in Israel. *Developmental Medicine and Child Neurology, 43*(4), 261–268.

Henderson, C. M. (2004). Genetically-linked syndromes in intellectual disabilities. *Journal of Policy and Practice in Intellectual Disabilities, 1*(1), 31–41.

Israeli Knesset Center for Research and Study. (2006). Children in the Bedouin community—The present situation. Jerusalem, Israel.

Jackson, A. P., McHale, D. P., Campbell, D. A., Jafri, H., Rashid, Y., Mannan, J., et al. (1998). Primary autosomal recessive microcephaly (MCPH1) maps to chromosome 8p22-pter. *American Journal of Human Genetics, 63*(2), 541–546.

Kesher Organization (The Organization of Special Families in Israel). (2011). *Special families in Israel: A collection of selected data and issues for Family Day*. Jerusalem, Israel.

Kofman, O., Berger, A., Massarwa, A., Friedman, A., & Abu-Jaffar, A. (2004). Long-term effects of toxic exposure to pesticides on cognitive process in children. In Conference proceedings, *Psycho-social challenges of indigenous societies: The Bedouin perspective*. Beer-Sheva, Israel: Ben-Gurion University of the Negev.

Lithwick, H. (2002). *Policy guidelines for rejuvenation of the Bedouin villages*. Jerusalem, Israel: The Center for the Study of Social Policies in Israel.

Lubetzky, H., Shvarts, S., Merrick, J., Vardi, G., & Galil, A. (2004). The use of developmental rehabilitation services. Comparison between Bedouin and Jews in the south of Israel. *Scientific World Journal, 15*(4), 184–192.

Manor-Binyamini, I. (2005). *An evaluation of an multidisciplinary training program for professionals working with special needs children in the Bedouin community*. Research Report. This research is part of a post-doctoral report. Beer-Sheva, Israel: The Department of Education and the Department of Social Work, Ben-Gurion University of the Negev.

Manor-Binyamini, I. (2007). Special education in the Bedouin community in Israel's Negev region. *International Journal of Special Education, 22*(2), 109–118.

Manor-Binyamini, I. (2010). The prevalence and characteristics of psychiatric disorders among adolescent Bedouin with mild-moderate intellectual disability. *International Journal of Special Education, 25*(2), 26–33.

Mazawi, A. E. (1997). *The system of education and psychological counseling services in the education system in Israel: Implications for the diagnosis and treatment of children with learning disabilities in Arab society*. Jerusalem, Israel: Addendum to the report of the Committee for Examining the Realization of the Abilities of Pupils with Learning Disabilities, The Ministry of Education, Culture and Sports and the Ministry of Science.

Morad, M., Morad, T., Kandel, I., & Merrick, J. (2004). Attitudes of Bedouin and Jewish physicians towards the medical care for persons with intellectual disability in the Bedouin Negev community. A pilot study. *Scientific World Journal, 13*(4), 649–654.

Muir, W. J. (2000). Genetics advances and learning disability. *British Journal of Psychiatry, 176*, 12–19.

Naon, D., Morgenstern, B., Shimael, M., & Veriblis, D. (2000). *Students with special needs: Evaluation of needs and coverage by services*. Jerusalem, Israel: The National Insurance Institute and Joint-Brookdale Institute.

Ornoy, A. (1998). Professor Ornoy's talk at the Knesset Committee for HagilHarach, 5.5.1998. Parents Committee for Special Education in the Arab Sector in the Negev (Ed.). (2000). *Position paper: Special education in the Arab sector in the Negev: From discrimination to affirmative action*. Jerusalem, Israel.

Sarid, Y. (1999). Minister Sarid's response to member of Knesset Barakkah's parliamentary question, 4/11/99. Jerusalem, Israel.

Shatil Organization for Social Change. (2002). *Special education in Arab society in Israel— A profile of institutional discrimination*. Jerusalem, Israel.

The Forum of Ben-Gurion University for the Advancing of Bedouin Children with Special Needs and The Ministry of Education. (2003, July). *Building an educational campus and rehabilitating Bedouin children with special needs*. Beer Sheva, Israel.

The Ministry of Education, Culture and Sports' Committee for Examining the Bedouin Education System in the Negev. (1998). A report commissioned by Zvulun Hammer, the Minister of Education, Culture and Sports, and submitted to the Ministry's management. 16/1/98.

Turnbull, A., & Turnbull, R. (2001). *Families, professionals, and exceptionality: Collaborating for empowerment* (4th ed.). Upper Saddle River, NJ: Merrill Prentice Hall.

Wisel, A., Talachmi, A., Kabaha, W. (2000). *Evaluation of the needs of students in the special education system in the Arab Sector—Perspectives of the school principals, teachers, experts in the therapeutic professions and parents*. Shefa-Amr, Israel: Agudat Hagalil, the Nationwide Arab Association for Research And Health Services (The Ministry of Education, Culture and Sports, 1998).

Chapter 7
Collaboration Between Professionals and Parents of Children with Disabilities in the Bedouin Community: A Phenomenological Case Study

We Make the Road by Walking.

(Horton and Freire 1990)

In this chapter, I have sought to give voice to the professionals working with Bedouin children with disabilities and their parents, as well as to the parents of Bedouin children with disabilities, whose voices have not been heard up until this point in the study.

This chapter is based on the premise that research is one of the best tools that societies can use to methodically expand the available body of knowledge, in order to better inform professionals working in the field (Arzubiaga et al. 2008). The research presented in this chapter is based on a phenomenological case study conducted in 2007, in which I attempted to understand the perceptions and the ways in which parents of children with disabilities in the Bedouin community and the professionals who treat these children comprehend and define both parenting and the concept and practice of collaboration in the school.

Choosing this research approach allowed us to focus on a single case as a closed system which is limited in scale—a "bounded system" (Stake 1997, p. 406). The advantage of the phenomenological approach is in allowing the researcher insight into the intersubjective world (neither the objective nor the subjective world), which is to say, the world that people have in common. In this particular case, the professionals and the parents share a world which they created, but at the same time, it is a world of imposed constraints, defined by the social and cultural structures created by the people who came before them. The phenomenological study presented here sought to reflect and reveal the perspectives of the observed individuals and the manner in which they defined, understood, and interpreted their respective—professional or parental—worlds.

In adopting this research method, I relied on two assumptions. The first was that case studies allow for a thorough analysis of a social unit or a phenomenon (Paton 2002), within a set of limits defined by the time, the place, and the participants. The second assumption was that the case study format would allow for the exploration of the unique culture of the Bedouin community.

I. Manor-Binyamini, *School-Parent Collaborations in Indigenous Communities: Providing Services for Children with Disabilities*, DOI 10.1007/978-1-4614-8984-9_7, © Springer Science+Business Media New York 2014

7.1 Methodology

The study population included 60 participants, 30 of whom were professionals working with children with intellectual disabilities in the Bedouin community, and the other half, parents of Bedouin children with intellectual disabilities. The reason for choosing this particular study population was that intellectual disability was— and still is—the only type of disability diagnosed in the Bedouin sector. Correspondingly, the only special education schools that exist in the Bedouin sector are for children with intellectual disabilities (for further details, see Chap. 6).

Regarding the professionals, this was a diverse study population, representing various fields and disciplines. Education professionals included principals, educators, and teachers; the welfare professionals were social workers; and from the paramedical field—physiotherapists. Some live in permanent settlements and some live in unrecognized villages; half of the professionals hold a BA and the other half have an MA degree; they all had worked with children with intellectual disabilities in the Bedouin community, and their level of experience ranged from 5 to 18 years (for more details, see Manor-Binyamini 2008a).

Regarding the selection of parents of children with intellectual disabilities (30), half lived in permanent settlements and the other half in unrecognized villages. The age of the parents ranged from 27 to 70 years. The number of children with disabilities per family ranged from two children to five children with disabilities, of these, 60 % of the children had medium-to-severe intellectual disabilities, and 40 % had mild intellectual disabilities (for more detailed information, see Manor-Binyamini 2008b).

7.2 Research Tools, Process, and Data Analysis

7.2.1 Background for the Research

The importance of the subject of collaboration and its examination first arose in focus groups held during a multidisciplinary training program for professionals working in the Bedouin community: a total of 48 professionals, Bedouins and Jews from diverse areas of expertise, participated in these focus groups. This training program was the first of its kind in Israel, in that it brought professionals from various disciplines and from different cultures in order to learn together. This framework created a space for an open dialogue of collaborative learning (Manor-Binyamini 2005). Within this collaborative learning space, the issue of working with parents of children with disabilities in the Bedouin community emerged repeatedly.

7.2.2 Personal Interviews

In the second phase of the study, in order ensure cultural and professional perspective and a theoretical understanding of the components of collaboration, semi-structured interviews were held with 30 professionals who represent significant informants. The interviewees were selected from the focus groups. The interview questions were based on issues raised in the focus groups.

At approximately the same time, a meeting was held with officials from one of the welfare offices in the Negev, and a decision was reached about which parents would be asked to be interviewed as part of the study. After completing the interviews with the professionals, 30 semi-structured interviews were held with parents of children with intellectual disabilities; the interview questions were based on the questions presented to the professionals.

Interviews with professionals were conducted by the researchers, whereas interviews with the parents were conducted by a Bedouin student who was completing the final stages of his MA degree in Educational Counseling with a focus on special education.

The main reason for choosing the interview format as the main tool for the research was that a face-to-face interaction is considered a valid and empowering way to work cross-culturally (Carpenter 2005). These interviews provided some clear indicators/principles of effective practice when working in a range of settings with indigenous parents of children with disabilities.

In addition to the interviews, I spent hundreds of hours observing a variety of activities in the daily lives of families of children with disabilities in the different tribes, in the permanent settlements, in the unrecognized villages, and in the special education schools.

7.2.3   Data Analysis

The data analysis process included three phases: (1) the open encoding phase, (2) the mapping phase, and (3) the "translation" phase.

1. The open encoding phase comprised a careful reading of all the data material collected, including all the notes and observations made, and the implementation of the Strauss and Corbin system (Strauss and Corbin 1990), by examining each line of the transcribed interviews and asking the question: what is the theme, the main topic of this line? This analysis identified 79 units, relating to all the research questions.
2. During the second analysis phase, the mapping phase, the units were sorted and combined into broader themes, based on connections found between the units, while grouping the units together (sorting them into units and subunits). Sorting was done according to the frequency with which the characteristic was mentioned and according to the degree to which the characteristic was considered significant (vs. incidental). The themes presented in the following sections of this chapter are those with the highest levels of prevalence.
3. The third analysis phase consisted of "translating" selected themes raised by the parents and professionals into behavioral dimensions that were either exhibited by or expected from the professionals.

7.2.4 *Trustworthiness/Validity*

Reliability was verified through the use of a variety of strategies, in order to increase the reliability of the study. These strategies included verbatim transliteration of all study materials, rechecking of research findings' codes, not only by the researcher and the research assistant, but also by an external researcher. The method of Apparent Validity was also employed: towards the end of the study, the findings were presented separately to the professionals and to the parents interviewed. Feedback from the professionals and the parents confirmed Apparent Validity.

7.3 Findings

The findings are presented here in two sections: first, the findings regarding the professionals, followed by the findings regarding the parents. In each section, the findings are presented according to themes corresponding to the two research questions (parenting and collaboration) and the decreasing frequency of the interviewees' responses.

7.3.1 *Professionals*

7.3.1.1 Professionals' Views on Parenting

Three themes were identified as representing the perceptions of the professionals regarding the parenting of children with intellectual disabilities: (1) the difficulty of raising a child with intellectual disabilities in the Bedouin community, (2) shame/abandonment or denial of the child's existence, and (3) parental resources.

Theme 1: *The difficulty of raising a child with intellectual disabilities in the Bedouin community*. According to the perceptions of 100 % of the professionals, raising a child with disabilities in the Bedouin community is more difficult than in other communities. Within this theme, the following issues were raised. Language difficulties were mentioned in relation to the scarcity of professionals who speak the Arabic language, as in the case of speech therapists, which was mentioned by all of the professionals. Accessibility difficulties regarding location and transportation: the professionals mentioned accessibility difficulties that parents, especially those who live in unrecognized villages, have to deal with, as different tribes often reside in remote areas. Additionally, women, as well as most men do not drive, and do not own private cars, so they depend on private or public transportation, and the stops where passengers are picked up are often located very far from the settlements of the tribes. In addition, professionals noted that a basic difficulty stemmed from the lack of precise information about the child's disabilities, which made it difficult to provide the proper type of support that parents needed. All of the professionals emphasized a lack of information regarding complex disabilities, knowledge of the definitions of the types of intellectual disabilities, their characteristics, and the ways in which they are expressed developmentally. Additionally, there is, in their opinion, a lack of knowledge of methods, teaching techniques, and possible adjustments applicable for this particular student population. As one social worker stated: "…A social worker must have the knowledge in order to understand the child's disability…."

The majority of the interviewees talked about the fact that in the Bedouin community, almost all of the disabilities are defined as an "intellectual disability." With the exception of deafness, there are almost "no children with any other types of disability," for example, mental disorders, behavioral disorders, or autism. This situation is reflected in the type of therapeutic frameworks available: there are three schools in the Bedouin sector whose population is defined as having an intellectual disability, but there is no appropriate framework for children with any other type of disability. One social worker noted: "If I, in my capacity as social worker, want to ensure that a Bedouin child with autism receive the proper care, I have to send the child to a Jewish school, which in turn creates other problems." In the opinion of the professionals, there is a need for an officially established support system. The lack of knowledge makes it difficult, they claimed, to help the parents in raising their children.

Theme 2: Shame, abandonment, or denial of the child's presence. The majority of the professionals (90 %) expressed the idea that parents perceive their parenting in terms of shame, abandonment, or denial of the child's presence. They offered various reasons for this, among them the fact that a child with an intellectual disability is perceived as dishonoring the family and the parents' reputation in the community. Parents tend to be ashamed of the miserable condition and appearance of the child with an intellectual disability, or perceive the child as marked by misfortune. As one educator noted, "children with intellectual disabilities in the Bedouin community are perceived by the parents as pitiful and as having an especially unluckydestiny, compared to the other siblings in the house."

These perceptions change the role of the parent, in the opinion of the professionals, and instead of caring for the daily needs and personal interests of the child, the parents focus on upholding the family name. This preoccupation with the family's reputation, claims the professionals, creates shame and unwillingness on the part of the parents to reveal the child to the community. One of the principles related the following.

> The Bedouin community is characterized by strong family ties which are manifested by the parents' constantly worrying about their children in every aspect, except when the family's reputation is at stake. Then the child's condition becomes irrelevant, overshadowed by the stigma and shame etc., associated with the child's condition… and here parental roles change, from concern for the personal interests of the child to upholding the family name.

Several of the social workers and physiotherapists interviewed mentioned another way that parents have found to deny the presence of a child with intellectual disability. They had witnessed cases in which the parents abandoned their special-needs children at the hospital, and denied that they ever had "such a child."

Professionals explained the various reactions of parents by referring to the family's religious beliefs. The religion of the Bedouins, which is based on the Islamic tradition, may lead some parents to accept "fate" and to come to terms with the child's disability, perceiving it as a state that depends on God's will and one that they cannot change. The role that religion plays for the family can be crucial, because it serves as a basis for their interpretation of the child's disability. It is important to understand that in the Bedouin community, the tenets and customs that guide the family are embedded in the culture itself.

Theme 3: *Parental resources*. According to the perceptions of 80 % of the professionals, the issue of parental resources is central to understanding their parenting behaviors. The most fundamental resource is the capability to support the child and his or her needs on a daily basis, in the sense of demonstrating awareness of the child's needs and a great willingness to invest time and effort in caring for the child. In the words of one of the educators:

> To support the child, to understand his difficulties, his rights, and the appropriate treatment for him requires a lot of effort, insight, and awareness on the parent's part, because without the effort and the tenacity, the parent wouldn't even have the strength to cope with the hassles, and without the awareness, the parent wouldn't have the mindset to worry about tests and treatments and special needs...

Along with what is said on this subject, according to the perceptions of the professionals, we can consider parenting in Bedouin society on a time axis: most of the professionals spoke in terms of "then" and "now," they noted that there were significant changes in Bedouin society regarding children with disabilities. These changes are expressed, according to their perceptions, in that parents nowadays are more open to collaboration, more concerned and show a greater interest in the care and the development of their children with disabilities.

7.3.1.2   The Professionals' Definition of Collaboration

How do the professionals define collaboration? Let me begin by noting that three professionals out of the 30 interviewees indicated that there was no collaboration between parents and professionals, because parents don't send their child to school. Hence, the analysis presented here is based on input from the 27 remaining professionals. Interviewees discussed two themes, which illustrate that collaboration with parents is an essential and fundamental part of their work. The first theme addresses the goals of the collaboration with the parents, namely, promoting their child's welfare; the second theme, unlike the first, related to the goal of strengthening and enhancing this collaboration between parents and professionals. In other words, the focus of the second theme is on the parents rather than on the child.

Theme 1: *The goal of the collaboration*. For most of the professionals, the purpose of collaborating with the parents was to agree on and set in motion a plan of action for the child's benefit. To realize this goal, the professionals identified three objectives.

A. *The need to increase parents' awareness of their children's basic needs.* According to the perceptions of the professionals, the parents are responsible for ensuring that the child is able to receive the required support services, but they need to understand the child's needs and be informed not only about the kind of support services available, but also about how to access them. The experts claimed in their interviews that instead of trying to convince parents to change their opinions and their beliefs, the professionals should refer to themselves as "interpreters or translators" of the approaches and resources available in the special education community, and as instructors who respectfully offer the family support services, which the family may then choose to use or reject. According to the professionals, when they serve as translators and interpreters of the existing practices, they can learn about the beliefs and culture of the family. Only then can a meaningful dialogue begin.

B. *Exhausting the child's rights.* Professionals perceived themselves as assisting parents to implement the rights to which child is entitled by law, for instance, obtaining equipment such as a cart or a walker, or receiving an implant for a hearing impaired child. One of the educators described the following situation.

> In my work, I encountered students who did not have eyeglasses, writing tools, or folders, and the parents were unwilling to purchase those things for them. There was one student with a mild intellectual disability, who was also blind, but she sat at home, she didn't have her blind person's card. There were some parents who didn't know their children's rights, children who were visually impaired or had other problems.

Additionally, professionals emphasized the importance of providing the parent with the necessary information. Thanks to this, one student who had been staying at home was finally enrolled in an educational framework. A social worker commented:

> I once got a report about a family of a girl with special needs. Trying to contact the family, I at first came across a great deal of suspicion and distrust from the parents. The parents were not providing their daughter with the proper care; she did not receive the necessary medical treatment and was not brought in for her follow up appointments at the Child Development Institute. It was my impression that the parents had no and no awareness or understanding of the child's condition and her disability. They saw the situation as a decree of God, and did not think that they could do anything about it. I spent a lot of time, conducted many home visits, gave the family a great deal of support and many explanations, and informed them of their child's rights, the importance of the treatments and, later, placement in an appropriate educational framework. The parents received thus both mental and financial help, and cooperated with me.
>
> The girl went back to therapy at the Child Development Institute; the parents bought her the rehabilitation equipment, and took her to the meeting with the placement committee. She now attends the appropriate special needs educational framework. And now the parents keep in constant contact with me, and come into my office to consult about other matters as well.

The professionals repeatedly emphasized that if a parent must decide between finding shelter and food or meeting and collaborating with the professionals, the parent would obviously take care of the first before attending to the second.

C. *Maintaining contact with the parent.* Professionals noted that to ensure the child's ongoing and proper care, it is necessary to maintain continuous contact with the parent. This is achieved by forging and strengthening the relationship with the parent. The professionals' objective, thus, is to make sure that they don't lose contact, which may become a frustrating exercise, in cases when the parent does not respond to the contacting attempts. Most of the professionals stressed how important it is not to give up, and to think of ways to create further dialogue with the parent.

Theme 2: *The goal of strengthening the collaboration.* Most of the professionals defined collaboration by what they do in their day-to-day work in order to strengthen the collaboration on the part of the parents. The focus of this theme is the work they do with the parents themselves, for instance, including the parents in the educational practice, inviting parents to attend meetings and school events; providing guidance to the parents on how to work with the child at home, coordination between and integration of the work being done at the school and the care provided at home; running workshops for parents and teachers; supporting the parents, expressing understanding and awareness of the parents' needs; and coordinating expectations. A principal of a special education school noted:

> Every organization must find its own method, language, and attitude through which it can maintain constant contact with the parents and thus create this collaboration. I make every effort to involve the parents at the school; we engage them any way we can.

7.3.1.3   "Translation" of Findings into Behavioral Dimensions: Skills and Strategies Used by Professionals to Work in Collaboration with Parents

Analysis of the behavioral dimension was intended to identify the interpersonal skills and the strategies employed by professionals in order to work in collaboration with the parents. The findings of this section are presented separately for skills and for strategies.

7.3.1.3.1   Skills Employed by Professionals

The skills used by professionals to facilitate collaboration with parents were divided into two themes, according to the professional's particular objective: (1) skills for getting to know the parents and (2) skills for containing the parents.

Theme 1: *Skills for getting to know the parents.* According to the perceptions of 100 % of the professionals, getting to know the parents has to include becoming acquainted with their culture and environment. Therefore, the entire process has to occur in the parent's own environment, so as to allow the professional to learn about the family's background, understand the values and codes of the family, become familiarized with the tribal or other interpersonal struggles, and in this manner find a common language with the family. Learning how to respect the parents' culture according to the family's own point of view is also necessary. Such learning does not end with knowing to which tribe the family belongs; this is not the key to collaboration. Respecting the culture begins with the effort to recognize each tribe and family and its individual characteristics. The professionals repeatedly mentioned that one must invest time, special time, and a lot of time, to get to know the parents and their environment.

Theme 2: *Skills for containing the parent*. According to the perceptions of 98 % of the professionals, the skills employed in the effort to contain the parents emotionally include listening, understanding, patience, and tolerance for the process that the parent goes through. In the words of one educator: "one should follow the timeline of the parent and the family, and that means not to pressure the parent and just to be the parent." The following anecdote was related by a teacher.

> I remember once, when I was the homeroom teacher, and I was constantly following up with a psychologist who would come to the school. At that time, I was also the coordinator of special education at the school. A parent came in yelling at us, demanding to know why we had sent him a form to sign, by which he was supposed to agree to send his son to a psychologist. "My son is not crazy," he yelled, "he has a good head on his shoulders and he has a brain…". And so, he went on shouting. I asked him to calm down, and then we sat and talked privately in a quiet room. I explained to him the role of the psychologist and the difference between a psychologist and a psychiatrist. I explained to him about his son's condition and his difficulties in school and what would become of him if we did not help him. I explained the process of providing support and how it requires a psychological assessment, in order to test for other conditions, and that in addition, we run diagnostic tests at the school. The father understood, calmed down, and signed the form.
>
> After that, the child was tested, and was found eligible for additional tutoring time, and after nearly a month, I met with the father again, and he was pleased with what had happened. One of the skills is to accompany the parents while taking care not to reinforce any negative feelings and to avoid entering into a conflict that you then cannot get out of. It is very important to find the time to meet with the parents, even if they do not keep to the schedule that was set. It's vital to seriously address the issue that made the parents come to speak to us in the first place, and to try to understand the goal of this visit, and not to forget the emotional aspect that the parents bring along with them.

According to the perceptions of the professionals, when parents feel that the professional is listening and attentive to their particular priorities at each stage of the support, the professional can become a partner who the parents can trust, which is the basis that enables the collaboration between them.

7.3.1.3.2 Strategies Employed by Professionals

What were the strategies employed by the professionals to encourage the parents' collaboration? Within the answers to this question, three themes were identified: (1) familiarity with the religion and clergy, (2) involving the existing multidisciplinary team of the school, and (3) modeling of collaboration.

Theme 1: *Familiarity with the religion and the clergy*. In the interview responses, 85 % of the professionals talked about "using religion," in the sense of being familiar with the religion and the clergy, and appealing to clergy in order to resolve difficulties, address the unique needs of the child, and sometimes to help address the parents' needs as well. One of the teachers expressed the following opinion.

> Not all meetings have to be only between a teacher or a member of the school team and the parent; you can also hold meetings with some other person who the parents trust, such as a member of the cultural community, the family, or the tribe. For example, a cleric might have a valuable contribution to the collaboration between parents and professionals. I think that the professionals constitute the formal support services system, while the family, community, and tribe constitute the informal support system in the Bedouin society, and are therefore very important.

According to the perceptions of the professionals, interventions that recruit the people who are already part of the parents' natural support network are most likely to succeed. Hence, it is important to meet the clerics who are significant to the parents and involve them: the intervention must be based on the parents' natural support network, in this case the help of religious leaders from the community.

Theme 2: Involving the existing multidisciplinary team of the school. According to the perceptions of 70 % of the professionals, involving the entire multidisciplinary team at the school in the work that is being done with the student is essential for the existence of collaboration with parents. This theme includes the following categories: collaboration for the purpose of Individual Educational Programs, collaboration for the purpose of diagnosing and evaluating the student, collaboration for the purpose of overall student care. Many of the professionals distinguished between the Individual Educational Programs and student care. According to them, care is responding to the needs of the student which are not being met at home and/or at school, anything related to everyday life and survival needs, such as diapers. For instance, one teacher brought diapers to school each morning, and diapered a girl who would arrive at school smeared with feces. Others told of administering medication to children whose parents do not follow the necessary course of treatment and of bringing food for students who come to school without lunch.

Most of the professionals mentioned collaboration for the purpose of Individual Educational Programs. These meetings are held at the beginning of the school year and sometimes also at the end. Interviewees emphasized that what takes place at these meetings is mainly the sharing of information about each student. There is no discussion of the goals of the work with each student, the student's diagnoses, or the evaluation findings. According to the interviewees, there is a gap between policy-related statements and the actual implementation. Based on their training, professionals know the importance of multidisciplinary teamwork and collaboration, but they note that in practice, there is only one session in which they share information. This gap may explain the distinction that most of the professionals drew between Individual Educational Programs and student care.

Theme 3: Initiating and maintaining collaboration. According to the perceptions of 68 % of the professionals, it is up to the professionals to initiate and maintain the collaboration with the parents. One educator noted the following.

> The contact and the beginning of the collaboration with the Bedouin community, in my opinion, should be initiated by members of the education system and not by the parents, because I'm assuming that for those who did not come to see me, it's up to me to go see them. What I mean is that parents in the Bedouin community are unaware of the importance of the collaboration or the importance of planning for the future; the parents depend on us and on the message that we, as the system, pass on to them.

The professionals mentioned that the response of the professionals and of the school to the parents' different customs and behaviors is what produces either positive or negative results in terms of the parents' collaboration.

This theme included the following categories: first, "courting" the parents, and second, the behavior of the professionals. "Courting" the parents includes inviting them to school to attend meetings, school events, school trips, and observation of the student, among other suitable activities. Successful collaboration was described as follows, by a social worker: "a successful collaboration is reflected in the parent's response and presence after the invitation was extended," and thus, by one of the teachers:

> The parents maintain ongoing and constant contact with the school; it speaks to a "successful collaboration". This means that the professionals consider a successful collaboration to be one where they are able to maintain regular contact with the parents. This requires professionals to initiate contact over and over again; it requires many calls to encourage and persuade the parents; patience and persistence. This guideline was iterated by one of the principals thus: "contact the parent even ten times if you have to, just do not give up", and in the words of a social worker: "be tolerant and have the power that God gives those who have patience and believe."

Theme 4: Providing practical solutions to the everyday difficulties raised by parents. All of the professionals mentioned the issue of providing solutions to the child's everyday problems which the parents have to face. One example is the following story about helping a child with skin problems.

> …. This is one student who used to be in my class. A very nice girl, shy, introverted, insecure, and neglected. She used to come to school without food or pocket money to buy food at the school kiosk, and in addition she had a visible skin disease. Her hands and even her face were covered with dry spots, like tattoos, and that made the students stay away from her, because it was infectious.
>
> At first I approached her, took her aside for a lot of conversation and built up her trust, and in addition I gathered information about her, about the family. It turned out that her mother was the father's second wife, and the father was very neglectful, and didn't visit them at all. The mother was depressed and the family was on welfare through the local council. So I made a point of helping her in every way. I let her feel that I cared about her, treated her like the mother she couldn't have and involved the principal and the school counsellor in everything that happened. I invited her mother and together we took the child to a doctor to take a look at her skin. The doctor gave us information and a prescription, along with a referral to a dermatologist in Beer Sheva, and we started buying her ointment, sometimes with the principal's money, sometimes with my money, as long as she got help and was feeling well. In addition, I got her a dermatologist appointment and went with them to the medical examination, and reported everything to the welfare department, so that they would pay for the medication and place all the kids in that family in daycare in the afternoons, so that they would at least get some food.

Not easy (4, 13%)	Very difficult (21, 70%)	Very difficult especially for the Bedouins (5, 16%)

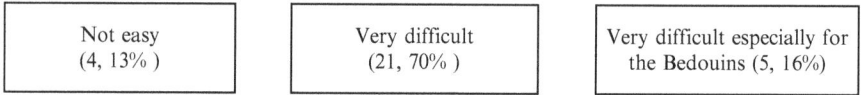

Fig. 7.1 A continuum of parents answers regarding their feelings of raising a child with a disability

7.3.2   Parents

The interviews with the children's parents were less informative than the interviews with the professionals, but numerous nonverbal behaviors were noticeable. Analysis of the nonverbal observations shows that the behavior which appeared most frequently and with greatest intensity was silence. Although the purpose of this study was not to examine nonverbal behaviors, the silence of the parents was deafening and is therefore significant and noteworthy.

A number of reasons may explain the informative difference between the professionals and the parents. First, the professionals are trained in giving interviews or talking in a way that requires them to be verbally eloquent regarding the field in which they work. Second, it is likely that the issue created a flood of emotions for the parents. Third, for some of the parents, this was the first time they were asked for their opinion and were able to share stories and information, and for others it was the first time they talked about being the parents of children with disabilities.

7.3.2.1   Parental Perceptions Regarding the Parenting of a Child with an Intellectual Disability in the Bedouin Community

All parents addressed this question. After the question had been posed, most parents took a deep breath; some lowered their heads and most of them kept silent a few seconds/minutes before answering the question. It was evident that the question was difficult for most parents. The question caused them to use very emotional language, unlike their replies to other questions. Analysis of 100 % of the findings raises two major themes in this area: emotions and feelings that come up when one is raising a child with an intellectual disability, and faith in God as a way of coping.

Theme 1: Emotions and feelings that come up when one is raising a child with an intellectual disability. Analysis of the observations of nonverbal behaviors showed that this question was emotionally difficult for the parents. Most of the parents were silent for a while before answering the question, and also, it seemed that for some of the parents, this was the first time they faced answering this question out loud, and were asked to define their perceptions. We can present the parents' answers to this question on a thematic sequence (Fig. 7.1):

Parents spoke with an emotional voice. Of the 30 parents interviewed, 22 (73 %) said they were angry and sad, 17 (56 %) of the parents talked about the pain of

raising a child with an intellectually disability, and 9 (30 %) of the parents emphasized that they love their child, but noted that they had "bad feeling," that they felt
uncomfortable in company due to feelings of shame. They explained that preferred
to avoid being among people, to stay at home with the child, and remain in the
safety of their own private space with the child suffering from the disability. Finally,
5 (16 %) of the parents mentioned that they had "no more strength left."

Theme 2: *Faith in God as a way of coping.* Analysis of the responses of 28 (93 %)
of the parents showed that the strength to cope with the challenge of raising a child
with an intellectual disability is based on faith. For example, 18 (64 %) of the parents indicated that faith strengthens them and gives them the mental energy to deal
with the day to day; 6 (21 %) of the parents said that "there is no choice, this is
God's decision"; 6 (21 %) mentioned that "we are religious and believe in God";
and 3 (10 %) others noted that "only God will help and forgive."

Some parents, in their response to this question, also addressed the child as well
as parenthood. Analysis of the data revealed a clear distinction between parents of
children with a mild intellectual disability and parents of children with a medium/
severe disability. Parents of children with mild disabilities perceived the child as a
"regular" child, as mentioned by 9 (30 %) of the parents, and 3 (10 %) parents said
that they treat this child as they do the others. In contrast, parents of children with a
medium/severe disability repeatedly referred to the child as "unfortunate, miserable," and expressed a wish that the child might get better, recover, and be a normal
child again, 10 (33 %) of the parents said over and over again: "We did everything
we could so that he would recover; the rest is in God's hands."

7.3.2.1.1   The Parents' Definition of Collaboration

In their responses to the question regarding collaboration, 6 (20 %) of the parents
indicated that there was no collaboration; hence, the analysis presented here is based
on 24 parents representing 80 % of the parents interviewed. The analysis of the
questionnaires of these 24 parents identified three main themes: (1) a continuum of
collaboration; (2) collaboration location; and (3) examples of a successful
collaboration.

Theme 1: *A continuum of collaboration.* Parents' answers to this question revealed
various degree of collaboration, which form a continuum. The following is a schematic presentation of this continuum (Fig. 7.2).

Parents who are not collaborative raised a variety of arguments; for example,
some said: "I don't want anything," another parent said: "I cannot give them [the
professionals] instructions," yet another said: "it doesn't matter to me—I was and
am doing fine." Another quote that reinforces this trend exhibited by the parents: "I
did not study after high school and I'm not a teacher and don't know anything about
special education, I'm fine and ready for anything." That is, the parents treat the
professionals' opinions as expert opinions with which they (the parents) are not
equipped to argue. Parents who were partially collaborative presented statements

Parents who are not collaborative	-------	Parents who are partially collaborative		Parents who are completely collaborative

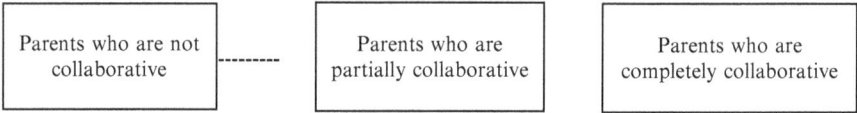

Fig. 7.2 A continuum of parents' collaboration

such as: "The most important thing is the child; I, as a parent, am less important." Among the parents who were completely collaborative, 9 (37 %) parents responded by describing a distinction between two concepts (without defining them) that the theoretical literature refers to as "involvement" and "collaboration." According to parents' perceptions, involvement means that the parents take part in activities that are a part of the child's education, such as meetings at school, consultations, training, and volunteer services. Collaboration includes maintaining a positive relationship, which is respectful and based on equality between the home and the school. This relationship includes mutual problem solving and joint decision-making. Regarding decision-making, for example, 14 (58 %) of the parents stated that the purpose of the collaboration is joint decision-making. The common goals, according to the perceptions of the parents, should be focused on the child, treatment issues, and should be implemented by law. Parents emphasized that they believed that parents of children with intellectual disability must be an active partner in identifying educational problems and finding solutions. They emphasize that the voice and the stories of the parents must be heard. Analysis of the findings indicated that some of the parents wished to enjoy collaboration as well as involvement and that some had had a positive experience with the school.

Theme 2: *Collaboration location*. Asked where they would like the collaborative work to take place, 22 (92 %) of the parents responded to this question, and most said their preferred location for the collaboration with the professionals was at their home or tent. They gave a variety of reasons for this request, for example, saving on travel expenses to the school or welfare office, and feeling uncomfortable away from home. These parents said they did not want to be exposed to others in their community, and wanted the process of diagnosis and support to take place at the home. According to the parents, there are two types of support that can be provided at the home: (a) instructions on how to work with the child at home, or alternatively, if the child attends kindergarten or school, instructions on how to continue the type of work done with the child in the educational setting in the home setting, so that the child would make progress; (b) directing the parents to the support services available for the child.

Theme 3: *Examples of a successful collaboration experience*. In response to the question regarding a successful collaboration experience, 2 (7 %) of the parents indicated that they had no successful experience of collaboration; another parent said he could not remember, 8 (27 %) of the parents said they had a number of successful experiences of collaborations, and 7 (23 %) other parents said they had experienced many collaborations with a successful outcome. Altogether, there were

12 (40 %) successful instances of collaboration among the parents who participated in the study. Analysis of their stories found two issues that were pivotal for enabling a successful collaborative experience.

(a) Receiving assistance and suggestions for coping strategies from the special school. For example, a father spoke about a school project that aimed to provide information to parents in the special school.

This is an example about the school, they had a project, and invited us parents, along with the children, and listened to our needs and the children's needs on different subjects, and they wanted to know if we wanted knowledge about certain subjects (at the first meeting, of course). I looked around, a lot of parents came, they all came with their kids. It was the first time I ever saw so many retarded children together. This project was a good idea, they [the professionals] were trying to change some things around and add to the existing plan. They treated us, the parents, with respect. They treated us like the people who know their own child best, and know how to deal with him better than they did, and also, because we are the ones who live with the child after school is out.

(b) Providing the parent with information. In one example, informing parents of their rights led them to send their daughter, who had previously remained at home, to attend an educational framework. Another parent told of a struggle to attain safer transportation for the children, which was carried out by the parents in collaboration with the school's professionals, for the benefit of children.

I'll tell you a success story; we collaborated with the school so that there would be a chaperon on the school bus. Every morning the drivers would come to where the tribe lives to take my child to school, and there was never an adult accompanying them during this drive. That's against the "transportation safety" laws. On several occasions the children, were injured during the drive, hurt each other, or hurt themselves. I called the person in charge of transportation repeatedly—that helped for a day, and sometimes not at all. I finally turned to teachers and the school principal, and explained to them that this is their problem as well as ours, and that we all suffer from it. We, the parents, along with the school cooperated: we chose representatives and together we turned to The Ministry of Education. The response from The Ministry of Education came immediately; they addressed the problem quickly, but we did not find the proposed solution sufficient. In the end, we decided to take this to court. We won, and the children got what they deserve—a safe ride.

Another father told of obtaining the equipment required for his daughter, who is blind.

My daughter is almost completely blind. She goes to school but we did not buy her eyeglasses or other equipment that she needed, because we had no money. We didn't know she needed a special document attesting to the fact that she is blind; we didn't know she had any special rights. I'm not the only parent who didn't know the rights of his child. Her teacher had arranged a meeting. All parents received an invitation that included a detailed agenda for the meeting. At the meeting, there were tables with refreshments and drinks, there were professionals there, and they brought some aid devices. The meeting was successful. For instance, there were discussions about issues such as transportation to school from distant locations and about feeding the students who come from a socioeconomically disadvantaged background… And we made decisions : [we formed] an organization of parents of visually impaired and blind students, which included also parents of students with other problems, and organized food for the students; enrichment programs for visually impaired and blind students, and so on. All this has contributed greatly to my daughter's wellbeing, both at school and in life; she has come a very long way.

In telling their success stories, parents emphasized several components. The places where they had experienced successful collaboration constituted one component: 11 (37 %) of the parents mentioned school, 9 (30 %) of the parents mentioned the welfare offices to which they belong, and 7 (23 %) mentioned the Institute of Child Development (a department within the national health maintenance programs). Another aspect noted was the professional's area of expertise: 11 (37 %) of the parents mentioned the homeroom teacher, 9 (30 %) mentioned the social worker, 4 others mentioned the school principal (14 %), 5 (17 %) of the parents mentioned the physiotherapist, and 2 (7 %) of the parents mentioned the psychologist. Finally, the parents spoke of the type of functioning on the part of the parent that allows for a successful collaboration; during this part, the parents spoke about parental capabilities, such as a calm demeanor and the ability to listen.

7.3.2.2 "Translation" of Findings into Behavioral Dimensions: Skills and Strategies That Parents Expected from Professionals

7.3.2.2.1   Collaboration Skills That Parents Expect from a Professional Who Works with Their Child

Responding to a question regarding the type of behaviors they expected from the professionals, the 22 (73 %) parents who responded raised several themes. The analysis of the parents' answers raises two themes: (1) "being a decent human being" and (2) specific skills.

Being a decent person. In their replies, 22 (73 %) of the parents indicated that a professional should be "a decent person," and several different meanings were assigned to this term: 18 (60 %) of the parents indicated that the professional must have a big heart, 10 (33 %) of the parents mentioned that the professional should have a special kind of character, but did not specify what kind, 9 (30 %) of the parents noted that the professional must love his/her work, and 6 (20 %) of the parents mentioned that the professional must have a strong personality. According to the perceptions of the parents, trained professionals are not defined as experts solely because they are good at their respective areas of expertise, but because of their ability to "be a decent human being."

Specific skills. The answers to this question were varied and the parents presented a large number of skills. I will present the skills according to the frequency with which they were mentioned: 12 (55 %) of the parents expected a professional to be an expert, act professionally, and be professionally influential; 10 (45 %) of the parents expected the professional to demonstrate dedication to and faith in their work; 7 (32 %) of the parents emphasized "balanced" and "calm"—as important qualities; 5 (23 %) of the parents expected the professional to keep his/her promises; and 3 (14 %) parents expected a professional to be able to provide guidance and advice. Additional qualities and skills that were mentioned only once were forgiving; tolerant; accepting of others; having the ability to help, to share with the parents, and to preserve confidentiality and privacy; having integrity; being available; and a willingness to invest time.

7.3.2.2.2 Parents' Perceptions of the Work Patterns That Professionals Should Employ in the Course of the Collaboration

This question asked about the work patterns that the parents wanted the professionals to follow when working with them. One significant theme was raised over and over again: according to the perceptions of 30 (100 %) of the parents, listening is a key component of collaboration. (Analysis of the research findings showed a variety of work patterns, but as each of these work patterns was presented only by one parent it was impossible to identify a central theme; hence, I will not introduce them here).

Listening. One communication pattern that was raised during every interview, i.e., by 100 % of the parents, was listening. The reason for the repeated mention of this concept is that listening is the language of acceptance. Parents are tuned into what is called in the professional jargon "empathic listening," meaning "to listen in order to truly understand." For example, this is one parent's description of the type of listening that was desirable in the context of collaboration:

> … I want him to really listen, with his eyes, with his ears, with his head and heart, not just listen to what I am saying, but to feel what I am feeling, to understand my behavior, what I am not saying …

Another father added the following.

> The most important thing is that he should listen to me, to us. We know our children better than anyone else, and we know what's right for them. A lot of the time I feel that they (the professionals) don't listen, they fill their reports, they ask a lot of questions, they don't have any time.

To summarize this chapter, I will present a diagram of the research topics, the dimensions of parenting and collaboration, and the behavioral dimensions that are recommended for the professionals working in an indigenous community (Fig. 7.3).

Abu-Sa'ad (1999) argues that the time has come to allow the Bedouin community to be a part of the solution regarding its own educational problems. According to him, the way to improve the situation of the Bedouin society is through engagement. In the case of the education of children with disabilities, I suggest that the word *engagement* be replaced with the word *collaboration*.

7.4 Principles of Indigenously Inclined Collaboration

The principles of indigenously inclined collaboration introduced in this section were derived from the case study discussed in the previous part of this chapter as well as from the information and insights accumulated through the entirety of this book.

Special education professionals are equipped with several theory- and model-based intervention strategies acquired during their professional training, from which they derive their working principles for collaboration with parents. What happens, then, when the working principles of professional intervention are not suitable for the community in which they work and are inconsistent with the contextual boundaries and characteristics? In such cases, the professionals must have at their disposal

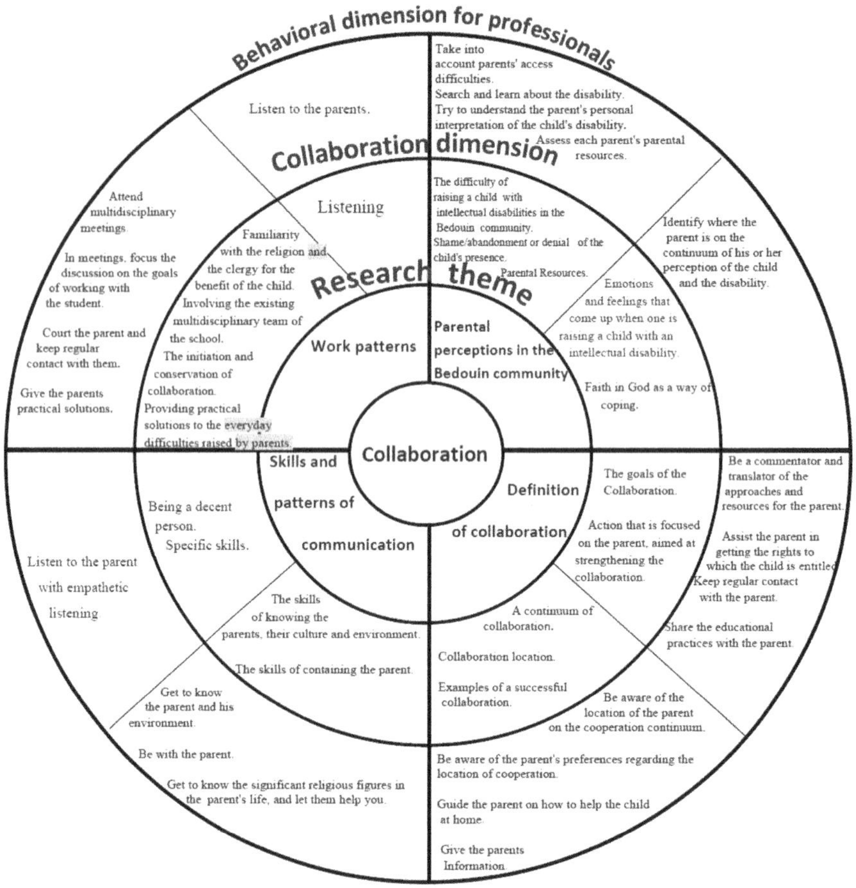

Behavioral dimension for professionals

Collaboration dimension

Listen to the parents.

Collaboration dimension

Take into account parents' access difficulties. Search and learn about the disability. Try to understand the parent's personal interpretation of the child's disability. Assess each parent's parental resources.

Attend multidisciplinary meetings.

Listening

In meetings, focus the discussion on the goals of working with the student.

Familiarity with the religion and the clergy for the benefit of the child. Involving the existing multidisciplinary team of the school. The initiation and conservation of collaboration. Providing practical solutions to the everyday difficulties raised by parents.

Research theme

Court the parent and keep regular contact with them.

Give the parents practical solutions.

Work patterns

Parental perceptions in the Bedouin community

The difficulty of raising a child with intellectual disabilities in the Bedoum community. Shame/abandonment or denial of the child's presence.

Parental Resources.

Identify where the parent is on the continuum of his or her perception of the child and the disability.

Emotions and feelings that come up when one is raising a child with an intellectual disability.

Faith in God as a way of coping.

Skills and patterns of communication

Collaboration

Definition of collaboration

Being a decent person.
Specific skills.

Listen to the parent with empathetic listening

The skills of knowing the parents, their culture and environment.

The skills of containing the parent.

Get to know the parent and his environment.

Be with the parent.

Get to know the significant religious figures in the parent's life, and let them help you.

The goals of the Collaboration.

Action that is focused on the parent, aimed at strengthening the collaboration.

Be a commentator and translator of the approaches and resources for the parent.

Assist the parent in getting the rights to which the child is entitled.

Keep regular contact with the parent.

A continuum of collaboration.

Share the educational practices with the parent.

Collaboration location.

Examples of a successful collaboration.

Be aware of the location of the parent on the cooperation continuum.

Be aware of the parent's preferences regarding the location of cooperation.

Guide the parent on how to help the child at home.

Give the parents Information

Fig. 7.3 Graphic representation of the research topics presented in this chapter

principles that will guide them as they seek to bridge the gap between the school culture and the indigenous culture. Using these principles will enable them to adjust their strategies to the culture of the client (in this case, the Bedouin parents of children with disabilities). Any other approach to collaboration is likely to create conflict and would require adjustments on the part of the parents, who are already experiencing high levels of stress. The purpose of the collaboration should be to bridge the gap between the two cultures, that of the special school and that of the indigenous community, in an attempt to spare the parents the experience of culture shock and out of awareness for the cultural blindness that the professional might have.

In this part, eight principles of indigenously inclined collaboration are presented, based upon the previous chapters and the case study discussed in the previous part of this chapter. Learning to become more responsive to different communities and cultures cannot be easily summarized in a checklist or in guidelines for appropriate practices to use with parents of children with disabilities in an indigenous community. The principles laid out here can, however, be used as a springboard for discussion. At the same time, they provide a backdrop from which to formulate new questions in a way that increases our understanding and our capacity to provide the best possible bridge to collaboration. The principles are presented here in an identical manner, referring to three elements: the subject of the principle, the assumptions behind it, and the goal of the principle.

7.4.1 Principle 1: Spend Time to Save Time

7.4.1.1 The Basic Assumption Behind the Principle

Since parents of children with disabilities constitute a population living with a dual identity—indigenous and disabled, they are an especially vulnerable group. Hence, collaboration in indigenous communities can exist only when the professionals understand and appreciate the struggle of the parent from the parent's point of view, that is, the point of view of the family, the community, and the ecological system to which the parent belongs. Working with parents of children with disabilities in an indigenous community requires a "wide angle lens," taking into account the large number of factors that affect the parents and the child; thus, we need to look at the big picture. It is only once we have looked at all the variables in the context of the parent as an individual, a member of an immediate and close-knit extended family, a member of a community, and a person with knowledge, can we begin to "zoom in" and focus on working with the parent.

7.4.1.2 The Goal of the Principle

A profound familiarity with the parent's contextual surroundings, a familiarity gained overtime, is a prerequisite for understanding the parent's worldview when encountering the professional/professionals, and it is the basis for the parent's collaboration or lack of collaboration. The time spent working respectfully and sensitively with parents from an indigenous community is a sound investment, and it may be the only way to ensure that the goals of the intervention are achieved.

7.4.2 Principle 2: Familiarity with the Communal/ Native Group and Recruiting Its Support

7.4.2.1 The Basic Assumption Behind the Principle

The communal or religious group constitutes a social support framework. People in indigenous communities care for each other, regardless of whether they are blood relatives. They support each other in different situations and help each individual cope, especially in a situation of crisis. Belonging to this group is an integral part of the daily life of the individual, and for that reason, the support of this group is important, because it can provide meaning for the parent, which in turn may help the parent cope during hard times.

7.4.2.2 The Goal of the Principle

In indigenous communities, the group framework to which the individual belongs extends beyond one's blood ties and clan, and it is an integral part of the individual's daily life. The professional's familiarity with this framework and the ability to recruit its support can empower the parent when coping with hardship. Even if the parent chooses not to share personal thoughts and feelings with the group members, the group framework may still give the parent the feeling that "we are here with you."

7.4.3 Principle 3: Indigenous Sensitivity

7.4.3.1 The Basic Assumption Behind the Principle

When working with parents of children with disabilities in indigenous communities, in addition to elements of cultural sensitivity and cultural competence, one requires indigenous sensitivity. The first step is to learn the indigenous history and the perceptions of the indigenous community, as well as the parent's perception of the disability. In addition, a familiarity and an understanding of the unique difficulties of the indigenous community to which the parent belongs are required, since these affect the collaboration of the parents. Indigenous sensitivity requires indigenous awareness, indigenous knowledge, indigenous competence, and indigenous sensitivity. It requires a flexible mind, an open heart, and a willingness to accept alternative perspectives.

7.4.3.2 The Goal of the Principle

Parents' perceptions of disability and support services are based on indigenous assumptions, rather than on universal truths.

7.4.4 Principle 4: Professionals as Cultural Mediators (Between Special School Culture and the Indigenous Culture)

7.4.4.1 The Basic Assumption Behind the Principle

The culture of the special school and the culture of the parents in indigenous communities are different (see Chap. 4). The culture of parents of children with disabilities in indigenous communities is characterized by several factors: existential challenges, i.e., poverty, poor living, and health conditions, and a heritage defined by subjugation; indigenous knowledge, i.e., culturally bound behaviors that affect interpersonal communication, and the meaning and causes of disability as perceived by the culture; indigenous psychology, which determines child rearing practices as well as the conceptualization of *development*, *goals*, and *time*. In contrast, the culture of the special school and/or of the professionals working in the school is characterized by a different set of factors: The school's culture represents the culture of the ruling establishment, professionals are viewed as experts, reliance on an exclusive source of knowledge, inflexible views due to "objective science", individual- (rather than community-) centered approach, embedded cultural expectations, and time constraints.

7.4.4.2 The Goal of the Principle

The role of the professional is to bridge the two cultures and to reduce the cultural shock that the parents may experience. Professionals working with parents in indigenous communities and cultures to which they do not belong find themselves in a position to bridge the gap between the two cultures. The goal is to avoid conflicts between the two cultures, conflicts which may harm the child's development and lessen the ability to respond to the child's needs.

7.4.5 Principle 5: Professional and Multidisciplinary Training for the Professionals

7.4.5.1 The Basic Assumption Behind the Principle

The chapters of this book indicate that collaboration between professionals and parents is a complex process, characterized by several basic components, and defined not only by certain structured professional obstacles, but also by the quality of the relationship between experts and parents. To facilitate this process, professionals should have the benefit of specific training, related to indigenous cultures in general and to the culture of the specific community where the professionals serve.

7.4.5.2 The Goal of the Principle

To collaborate with parents of children with disabilities in indigenous communities and bridge the gap between the two cultures, professionals need knowledge, skills, sensitivity, and awareness of indigenous variables. In other words, professionals need training, which can be provided before they begin working, as well as during their time working in special education schools in indigenous communities.

7.4.6   Principle 6: Expansion of the Role of the Professional

7.4.6.1   The Basic Assumption Behind the Principle

As noted earlier (in Chap. 1), parents of children with disabilities in indigenous communities have a wide variety of needs, including the need for more extensive support services, due to the unique characteristics of indigenous communities, among them, the high frequency of health risks; the elevated school dropout rates, and lack of financial resources.

7.4.6.2   The Goal of the Principle

Given that parents of a child with a disabilities in an indigenous community is in need of various support services, in addition to assistance in many existential, everyday needs, the most important work of the professional in the indigenous community may be the ability to provide parents with concrete support that addresses their everyday existential needs, such as providing clothing, school supplies, food, and transportation for their child.

7.4.7   Principle 7: A Discussion on the Effects That School Decisions Have on the Parent's Community and Environment

7.4.7.1   The Basic Assumption Behind the Principle

Societies have informal reward and punishment mechanisms. Society either looks favorably upon the behavior or attitude of the individual, or sanctions them, according to the degree to which they adhere to the boundaries that the community has set for itself. A parent acting in accordance with the conventions of the community and its boundaries would be welcomed and entitled to the community's support, whereas a parent who makes choices that do not correspond to the community's guidelines might be censured, depending on the degree to which the community's conventions were breached.

7.4.7.2   The Goal of the Principle

Helping the parent while demonstrating a profound regard for the effects that collaborative decisions could have on the parent's family, clan, and extended community will ensure that decisions and plans are made in accordance with the indigenous culture, knowledge, and values. Disregarding these effects jeopardizes the entire collaborative effort.

7.4.8   Principle 8: Learning from Success

7.4.8.1   The Basic Assumption Behind the Principle

Professionals working in indigenous communities with parents of children with disabilities experience success in their daily work. Experiences of professional success are important, because they provide orientation for further success; they reinforce the professionals' coping abilities and enhance their motivation to continue to cope with their professional challenges.

7.4.8.2   The Goal of the Principle

It is important to equip professionals with a theoretical background about indigenous cultures, emphasizing the method and importance of identifying experiences of success in their work, as well as ways to learn from these experiences.

References

Abu-Sa'ad, E. (1999). The Bedouin educational system is a changing social reality. In E. Peled (Ed.), *Fifty years of Israeli education* (pp. 1101–1111). Jerusalem: Ministry of Education.

Arzubiaga, A. E., Artiles, A. J., King, K. A., & Harris-Murri, N. (2008). Beyond research on cultural minorities: Challenges and implication of research as situated cultural practice. *Exceptional Children, 74*(3), 309–327.

Carpenter, B. (2005). Early childhood intervention: Possibilities and prospects for professionals, families and children. *British Journal of Special Education, 32*(4), 176–183.

Horton, M., & Freire, P. (1990). *We make the road by walking—Conversation on education and social change*. Philadelphia: Temple University Press.

Manor-Binyamini, I. (2005). *Evaluation of interdisciplinary training program for professionals who work with children with special needs in the Bedouin community—First operational year: 2004–2005*. Research report. [Research done as part of a post-doctoral paper and submitted to the members of the program's Steering Committee]. Israel: Department of Education at Ben-Gurion University. (in Hebrew).

Manor-Binyamini, I. (2008a). *Dimensions of collaboration between professionals and parents of intellectually disabled Bedouin children—Interdisciplinary aspect*. Research report. Jerusalem: The Shalem fund. (In Hebrew).

Manor-Binyamini, I. (2008b). *Dimensions of collaboration between professionals and parents of intellectually disabled Bedouin children—Parents' aspect*. Research report. The Robert H. Arnow Center for Bedouin Studies and Development. (In Hebrew).

Paton, M. Q. (2002). *Qualitative research and evaluation method*. Newbury Park: Sage.

Stake, R. E. (1997). Case study method in educational research: Seeking sweet water. In R. M. Jaeger (Ed.), *Complementary methods for research in education* (pp. 401–414). Washington, DC: American Educational Research Association.

Strauss, A., & Corbin, J. (1990). *Basics of qualitative research: Grounded theory procedures and techniques*. Newbury Park: Sage.

.

Index

I. Manor-Binyamini, *School-Parent Collaborations in Indigenous Communities:*
Providing Services for Children with Disabilities, DOI 10.1007/978-1-4614-8984-9,
© Springer Science+Business Media New York 2014

Printed in Australia
AUHW011601170420
326471AU00035B/355

9 781493 943739